Mosby's Guide to

WOMEN'S
HEALTH

A Handbook for
HEALTH
PROFESSIONALS

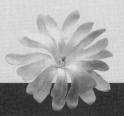

Mosby's Guide to

WOMEN'S
HEALTH

A Handbook for
HEALTH
PROFESSIONALS

TOLU OYELOWO, DC

Associate Professor
Chair, Diversity Committee
Northwestern Health Sciences University
Bloomington, Minnesota

EDITORIAL BOARD

Rosanna Urbano, RN, MSN, CRNP
Women's Health Nurse Practitioner
Nursing Faculty
Montgomery County
Community College
Blue Bell, Pennsylvania

Cynthia E. Neville, PT
Clinical Corporate Director of
  Women's Health Rehabilitation
Rehabilitation Institute of Chicago
Chicago, Illinois

Jenni Johnson Gabelsberg, DPT, MSc, MTC
Women's Advantage, Inc.
Women's Health Physical
  Therapy Clinic
Torrance, California

Mary Dockter, PT, PhD
Assistant Professor and Director
  of Clinical Education
University of Mary Program in
  Physical Therapy
Bismarck, North Dakota

MOSBY

ELSEVIER

MOSBY
ELSEVIER

11830 Westline Industrial Dr.
St. Louis, Missouri 63146

MOSBY'S GUIDE TO WOMEN'S HEALTH: ISBN: 978-0-323-04601-5
A HANDBOOK FOR HEALTH PROFESSIONALS
Copyright © 2007 by Mosby, Inc., an affiliate of Elsevier Inc.

Notice

Knowledge and best practice in this field are constantly changing. As new research and
experience broaden our knowledge, changes in practice, treatment and drug therapy may
become necessary or appropriate. Readers are advised to check the most current
information provided (i) on procedures featured or (ii) by the manufacturer of each
product to be administered, to verify the recommended dose or formula, the method
and duration of administration, and contraindications. It is the responsibility of the
practitioner, relying on their own experience and knowledge of the patient, to make
diagnoses, to determine dosages and the best treatment for each individual patient, and
to take all appropriate safety precautions. To the fullest extent of the law, neither the
Publisher nor the Author assumes any liability for any injury and/or damage to persons
or property arising out of or related to any use of the material contained in this book.
                                                                The Publisher

---

ISBN: 978-0-323-04601-5

Senior Editor: Kathy Falk
Senior Developmental Editor: Christie M. Hart
Publication Services Manager: Linda McKinley
Senior Project Manager: Kelly E.M. Steinmann
Designer: Andrea Lutes

Printed in the United States of America

The Publisher's policy is to use **paper
manufactured from sustainable forests**

Working together to grow
libraries in developing countries

www.elsevier.com | www.bookaid.org | www.sabre.org

ELSEVIER   BOOK AID
International   Sabre Foundation

Last digit is the print number: 9 8 7 6 5 4 3 2 1

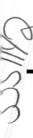

To My Mother
T.O.

Preface

Although women account for more physician office visits than men, most women receive diagnoses and treatments based on what has worked for men. Until recently, medical research has largely ignored many health issues important to women, and women have long been under-represented in clinical trials. Many health education programs have realized this inequity and have begun to incorporate women's health programs into their curriculum.

Mosby's Guide to Women's Health: A Handbook for Health Professionals will appeal to students and practitioners in the allied health professions. Although there are many women's health books and textbooks, most are medical textbooks designed for the gynecologist or obstetrician and provide far more detail than needed by the allied health student and practitioner. None of the medical texts discuss complementary and alternative medicine in any detail. Some provide insights into complementary and alternative choices and some even provide self-help protocols, but none provide information on as many conditions as this manual.

This manual is concise and organized for easy retrieval of information on women's health while providing firsthand information on traditional and natural health care management options. The conditions covered range from dysmenorrhea and endometriosis to cardiovascular health and osteoporosis. There is also a section on general hormonal health, with emphasis on the role of estrogen and estrogen derivatives in maintaining health and predisposing to disease. Given the impact of culture, spirituality, and domestic violence on the health of women, chapters on cultural considerations in women's health and domestic violence screening/referral are also included.

This book is:

Pocket-sized—It can fit in the pocket of a lab coat during clinics/rotations/examinations.

Consistent—The format is consistent throughout each chapter. All chapters that cover conditions are divided into the following subheadings:

> Description/definition of condition
> Who gets it?
> What are the causes?
> How is it diagnosed?
> Signs/symptoms
> Management
>> Traditional
>> Self-help treatments
>> Dietary management
>> Nutritional recommendations (vitamins, minerals, and herbs [where pertinent])
>> Adjunctive management
>> Chiropractic treatment

Multidisciplinary—A review panel includes physical therapists, nurses, and other rehabilitation professionals in the allied health fields.

Thorough—A wide variety of topics cover women's physical health, not just reproductive health.

Contents

1

Anatomy, Physiology, and Neurology

ANATOMY OF THE FEMALE GENITALIA

External Genitalia (Figure 1-1)

The external genitalia are bordered superiorly by the mons pubis, laterally by the labia majora, and inferiorly by the perineum.

The *mons pubis* is the fat pad covering the symphysis pubis (pubic bone), which is the anterior ring of the pelvic bone.

The *labia majora* are the two lateral borders of the vulva; they consist of skin, sebaceous glands, and adipose tissue and provide cushion and protection to the sensitive structures encased within the labia minora.

The *vulva,* also known as the pudendum, includes the labia majora (large lips), labia minora (small lips), clitoris, urethral and vaginal introitus, fourchette, fossa navicularis, vestibule, vestibular bulb, Skene's glands, Bartholin's glands, perineum, and hymen.

The *fourchette* is the band of mucous membrane that connects the posterior ends of the labia minora.

The *labia minora* are the two thin, sensitive internal lips of the vulva that enclose the vestibule at its superior borders and encase the clitoris. The anterior fold of the labia minora forms the prepuce or covering of the clitoris.

The *clitoris* is the small erectile tissue that is homologous to the male penis. It consists of two crura, a body, and a glans. The body consists of two fused corpora cavernosa approximately one inch long and extends from the pubic arch above to the glans below. The two crura are continuations of the corpora cavernosa and serve to attach them to the inferior rami of the pubic bones.

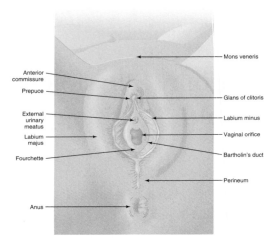

FIGURE 1-1 External genitalia. (From Hacker NF, Moore JG, Gambone JC: *Essentials of obstetrics and gynecology,* ed 4, Philadelphia, 2004, WB Saunders.)

The small, rounded glans is the distal end and consists of sensitive erectile tissue.

The *perineum* is the area below the vagina and above the anus.

The *anus* is the rectal opening.

The *hymen* is the thin, fibrous tissue that partially covers the vagina, leaving an opening for vaginal or menstrual discharge. It can be stretched or torn by sexual activity and sports activities. The size, shape, and degree of opening can vary greatly among individuals. This has been known to create challenges within cultural systems that erroneously use the state of the hymen as an assessment of virginity.

Internal Genitalia (Figure 1-2 and Figure 1-4)

The internal genitalia include the two ovaries, two fallopian tubes, uterus, vagina, and Bartholin's glands.

The *ovaries* are almond-shaped structures that function to produce the ova and the sex steroids.

The *fallopian tubes* (also known as the *oviduct*) are the locus of fertilization and extend from the fundus of the uterus to the ovary.

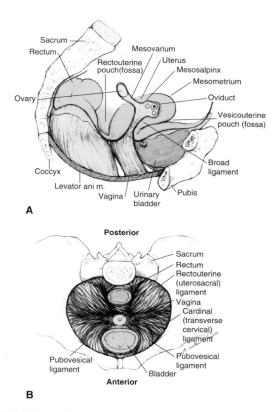

FIGURE 1-2 Internal genitalia. (From Mathers LH et al: *Clinical anatomy principles*, St Louis, 1996, Mosby.) *See also* Figure 1-4, page 6.

The *Bartholin's glands* are located on the inferior and lateral surface of the vulva; they open into the vagina and produce a thin mucus that helps to lubricate the vagina.

The *uterus* is a muscular, hollow, pear-shaped structure that nourishes and supports the embryo and developing fetus from the time that the fertilized egg is implanted.

The inner lining of the uterus is the *endometrium* and consists of blood-enriched mucous membrane. The outer fascia is mostly *peritoneum*.

The uterus consists of the *cervix,* the body, and the isthmus (neck). The most superior portion of the body is the fundus. It is situated in the middle of the pelvis, between the sacrum and the symphysis pubis, and is primarily supported by the pelvic diaphragm, two broad ligaments, two round ligaments, and two uterosacral ligaments.

The Breast (Figure 1-3)

The breast is both a milk producer and an organ of sexual stimulation. It consists of ductal tissue, glandular lobes, and fatty tissue. The tissues of the breast respond to stimuli from the ovarian hormones estrogen and progesterone and from other endocrine glands. These responses may result in milk production as occurs in the postpartum, swelling and tenderness during the premenstruum, or aberrations in growth patterns as seen in some malignancies. The brown, pink, or reddish area surrounding the nipple is the areola.

NEUROANATOMY

The *endocrine glands* are under the influence of the sympathetic, parasympathetic, and central nervous systems. Stimuli are mediated through the hypothalamus.

Vasomotor supply to the hypothalamic area is via the carotid and cavernous plexus from the superior cervical ganglia in front of the second and third cervical vertebrae.

Endocrine products reach their target areas via blood vessels that are controlled by the *vasomotor nerves* of the sympathetic nervous system.

Parasympathetic nerve supply to the uterus is via the inferior mesenteric plexus, with the nerves exiting from the sacral foramen. Sympathetic nerve supply to the uterus and ovaries is via the thoracolumbar spine. There are no known parasympathetic fibers to the ovaries.

Sympathetic nerve supply to the breasts is derived from the upper thoracic and midthoracic spines.

ARTERIAL AND VENOUS SUPPLY

Ovary

Blood supply to the ovaries is derived from the ovarian artery, which reaches the ovary through the infundibulopelvic ligament and the ovarian branch of the uterine artery.

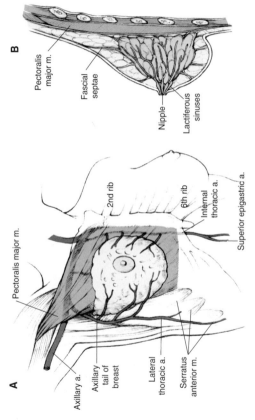

FIGURE 1-3 The female breast. (From Mathers LH et al: *Clinical anatomy principles*, St Louis, 1996, Mosby.)

Venous flow from the left ovarian vein is into the left renal vein.

Venous flow from the right ovarian vein is into the right inferior vena cava.

Fallopian Tubes

Blood supply to the fallopian tubes is via the ovarian and uterine arteries.

Venous flow from the fallopian tubes is into the ovarian and uterine veins.

Uterus (Figure 1-4)

Blood supply to the uterus is derived from the ovarian and uterine arteries. The uterine artery is derived from the internal iliac artery. The uterine venous plexus flows into the uterine vein and subsequently into the internal iliac vein.

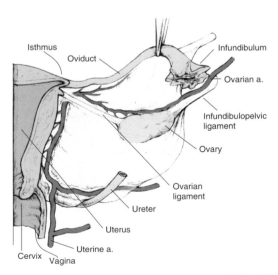

FIGURE 1-4 Blood supply to the uterus and vagina. (From Mathers LH et al: *Clinical anatomy principles,* St Louis, 1996, Mosby.)

Vagina

Upper. The vaginal artery and a branch of the uterine artery supply the upper vaginal vault, and the inferior vesical and middle rectal arteries send branches to the vaginal wall.

Lower. The internal pudendal artery supplies the vestibule and the lower vagina.

Venous return for the upper and lower vagina is via the vaginal plexus and the uterine plexus into the internal iliac vein.

Lymphatics

The ovaries, tubes, fundus, and the body of the uterus empty into the preaortic node (also known as the deep lumbar nodes).

The cervix and upper vagina empty into the sacral, hypogastric, and superior iliac glands.

The vulva and lower vagina empty into the superficial and deep inguinal nodes.

Table 1-1. Clinical Pearl.

Common Referred Pain Patterns	
Viscerosomatic pain from the	May refer to
Ovaries	T12 and the medial thigh
Fallopian tubes	T11 and T12
Uterus	T10-L1 and the lower abdomen
Cervix	S2-S4
Vagina	Low back and buttocks
Ureter and uterine ligaments	Across the lumbosacral area
Cervix	Sacral base
Rectum and trigone of the bladder	Sacral apex

From Clarke-Pearson DL, Dawood MY: *Green's gynecology: essentials of clinical practice,* ed 4, Boston, 1990, Little, Brown.

2

Estrogen Concepts

TERMINOLOGY

Xenoestrogens: Xeno = Foreign

Xenoestrogens are "foreign" estrogens, substances that are close enough in molecular structure to estrogen that they can bind to estrogen receptor sites with potentially hazardous outcomes.

Sources of xenoestrogens include plastics, pesticides, chemicals, and water systems.

Phytoestrogens: Phyto = Plant

Phytoestrogens are plant derivatives that have a similar structure to estrogen and can bind to the estrogen receptor sites. They are weaker endogenous estrogens and, through competitive inhibition, can prevent the receptor binding of more potent estrogens.

ESTROGEN

Estrogen is a broad term used to describe the predominant female hormone. Estrogen has three major derivatives:

- Estradiol–the primary form of estrogen before menopause
- Estrone–the primary form of estrogen after menopause
- Estriol–a byproduct of estrogen metabolism

Estrone and estradiol are created naturally in the steroidogenic pathways of the body (ovaries and adrenal glands). They are further metabolized by the liver and other tissues into approximately 40 metabolic products, called *metabolites*, one of which is estriol.

Many of the metabolites have important functions of their own. Examples include the catechol estrogens, liver metabolites formed from estradiol and estrone, which have a chemical structure that is part estrogen and part catecholamine. (Catecholamines are biologically active amines, e.g., epinephrine and norepinephrine derived from the amino acid tyrosine, which have marked effects on the nervous and cardiovascular systems, metabolic rate, temperature, and smooth muscle.)

Catechol estrogens have been shown to decrease the growth of some existing cancers,[1] inhibit abnormal growth of cardiac fibroblasts (thereby decreasing the risk of hypertension and myocardial infarction [MI]), and inhibit the action of leukotrienes[2] (hence decreasing inflammation, arthrosclerosis, and osteoporosis). In addition, catechol estrogens have antioxidant properties. Estradiol is the most potent of estrogens occurring naturally in the body. It is the primary hormone produced by the ovaries during the reproductive years. It is the primary hormone responsible for the menstrual cycle and also affects bone, blood vessels, heart, brain, and skin health. In its function intensity, estradiol is 12 times stronger than estrone and 80 times stronger than estriol.

Blood levels of estradiol before menopause are 40 to 350 pg/ml; in menopause, blood levels drop to less than 15 pg/ml. Ovaries are the predominant producer of estradiol, with the adrenal glands contributing approximately 4% and the placenta during pregnancy also contributing some.

The major source of estradiol in postmenopausal women is the conversion of estrone to estradiol by the enzyme aromatase, which is present in adipose cells.

The estradiol-to-estrone dual conversion works two ways. However, it does not work as effectively each way: 15% of estradiol is converted to estrone, but only 5% of estrone is converted to estradiol.

Conversion of estradiol to estrone takes place in the liver and other tissues; estrone is converted back to estradiol by the aromatase enzymes in fat tissue; but, with less being made by the ovaries, estrone levels still dominate in the menopausal woman. Because aromatase enzyme is present in fat tissue, there is increased conversion of androstenedione to estrone with increased body fat (i.e., there are benefits that come with adequate estrogen during menopause, but also problems that come with increased estrogen during menopause, such as increased risk of certain cancers). Estradiol is responsible for growth and female development. It increases the amount of fat in subcutaneous tissues, especially the breasts, thighs, and buttocks, and increases hip bone formation, resulting in the characteristic female skeletal development.

Estrogens work by crossing the cell membrane and attaching to estrogen receptors on the nucleus. Each type of estrogen has a different ability (receptor affinity) to stay attached to the receptor on the nucleus (nuclear retention). The stronger the receptor ability and the longer the nuclear retention time, the more potent the physiologic action of the estrogen. Estradiol has a nuclear retention time of 6 to 24 hours; estriol has a nuclear retention time of 1 to 4 hours.

Some of the known catechol estrogens are 2-hydroxyestradiol, 4-hydroxyestradiol, 2-hydroxyestrone, and 4-hydroxyestrone. Studies have shown that 2-hydroxyestradiol and estrone may decrease the growth of some existing cancers and inhibit abnormal growth of cardiac fibroblasts, the risk of which increases in postmenopausal women and which are associated with increases in hypertension, MI, and cardiovascular disease.

REFERENCES

1. Bradlow HL: 2-Hydroxyestrone: the good estrogen, *J Endocrinol* 150(suppl): S259–S265, 1996.
2. Alanko J et al: Catechol estrogens as inhibitors of leukotriene synthesis, *Biochem Pharmacol* 55(1):101–104, 1998.

3

Menstrual Cycle

The menstrual cycle occurs in four phases:

1. Preovulation
2. Ovulation
3. Postovulation (secretory phase)
4. Menses

The low levels of estrogen and progesterone that occur during menses trigger the secretions of gonadotropin-releasing hormone (GnRH) from the hypothalamus (Figure 3-1). GnRH stimulates the anterior pituitary to secrete follicle-stimulating hormone (FSH), which facilitates the development of the primary follicle in the ovary, estrogen synthesis, and secretion. Rising levels of estrogen cause the endometrium and breast tissues to proliferate and may contribute to the hypothalamic secretion of GnRH substrates, which facilitate the secretion of luteinizing hormone (LH) from the anterior pituitary. The surge of LH is the stimulus for ovulation. The remnant of the follicle, known as the yellow body or the corpus luteum, secretes progesterone and estrogen, which together prepare the endometrial lining for implantation. Progesterone in particular causes the endometrium to acquire nutrients that nourish the zygote if implantation occurs.

GENERAL CONSIDERATIONS

- The length of the menstrual cycle is 21 to 35 days, with most averaging 26 to 28 days.
- The duration of the secretory phase is relatively constant, averaging 14 days.

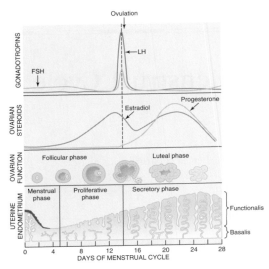

FIGURE 3-1 The hormonal levels during a normal menstrual cycle. (From Hacker NF, Moore JG, Gambone JC: *Essentials of obstetrics and gynecology,* ed 4, Philadelphia, 2004, WB Saunders.)

Technical Note
Subtracting 14 days from the length of the menstrual cycle should give an approximate date of ovulation. A woman with a menstrual cycle interval of 35 days can be expected to ovulate on or around the twenty-first day; a woman with a menstrual cycle interval of 23 days can be expected to ovulate on or around the ninth day.

- In the absence of fertilization, rising levels of estrogen and progesterone from the corpus luteum have a negative feedback effect on the anterior pituitary, causing it to "shut off" production of FSH and LH. The result is declining levels of FSH and LH, and a subsequent decline in the levels of estrogen and progesterone from the corpus luteum.

The blood vessels of the endometrium fail to be nourished; they die and are sloughed off as menstrual blood.

- If fertilization and subsequent implantation occur, the lining of the uterus changes its morphologic structure to become the decidua, which ultimately develops into the placenta. The decidua produces human chorionic gonadotropin (HCG), which nourishes and maintains the corpus luteum. The corpus luteum continues to produce progesterone, which in turn maintains the decidua in a "self-propagating" cycle. By the twelfth week, the placenta has formed and is self-sufficient.

- At birth, the ovarian follicles number approximately 600,000. At puberty, the number of ovarian follicles has declined to approximately 300,000, and by menopause it has declined to <30,000. The presence of large numbers of follicles at the beginning of puberty is essential for normal ovulatory cycles. The full maturation of one dominant follicle depends on the development of the support follicles, which secrete hormones such as estradiol, inhibin, and androgens, necessary for the appropriate functioning of the hypothalamic-pituitary-ovarian-uterine axis.

Clinical Pearl

Inadequate numbers or functioning of the support follicles may influence conditions such as polycystic ovary syndrome (PCOS) and premature ovarian failure.

SUMMARY

- Primary organs: hypothalamus, anterior pituitary, ovaries, and uterus. The hypothalamus produces GnRH, the anterior pituitary produces FSH and LH, and the ovaries produce estrogens and progesterone.
- *Onset:* For most girls, menarche begins at or around age 12, but it can start as early as age 8 and as late as age 16.
- The length of the cycle varies from 21 to 35 days, with an average of 28 days. Cycles occurring at 45-day intervals have been reported.

- Duration of flow varies from 2 to 8 days, with most averaging 4 to 7 days.
- Primary hormones of the first half of the menstrual cycle include FSH from the pituitary gland and estrogen from the ovaries. Primary hormones of the second half of the menstrual cycle include progesterone and estrogen from the ovaries.

Clinical Pearl

- *Secretions of GnRH from the hypothalamus are pulsatile. The pulses occur every 90 minutes. Alterations of this rhythm will hinder the production of FSH and LH from the anterior pituitary, which may cause amenorrhea or oligomenorrhea. Stress can induce GnRH arrhythmia.*
- *Progesterone is a thermogenic hormone and thereby elevates the basal body temperature (BBT). Assessment of BBT over the course of a cycle can provide guidance for natural family planning either as a method of birth control or to optimize fertility. The BBT elevates after ovulation and ideally remains elevated for approximately 10 days.*

Technical Note

The principal factor responsible for normal pubertal growth is insulin-like growth factor–I (IGF-I). Growth hormone exerts its action through the locally produced mediator, IGF-I; however, growth hormone can directly stimulate epiphyseal cartilage growth. Normal growth at puberty requires the concerted action of growth hormone, IGF-I, estrogen, progesterone, and the other sex steroids.

TERMINOLOGY

Adolescence–The period between puberty and adulthood.
Puberty–The phase of development typically between ages 8 and 16 when sexual maturation occurs, and the child becomes capable of reproduction.

Adrenarche–The phase of puberty marked by an increase in adrenal activity, pubic hair, and axillary hair.

Gonadarche–The phase of puberty marked by increased gonadal stimulation, primarily during sleep. There are no feedback mechanisms. The ovaries and uterus enlarge, the labia become more prominent, breasts increase in size, and body fat distribution begins to change.

Menarche–The first menstrual period.

Thelarche–The first stage of breast development.

Amenorrhea–Absence of menses.

Menorrhagia–Excessive bleeding or menstrual flow lasting longer than 7 days.

Metrorrhagia–Irregular bleeding or bleeding between cycles.

Menometrorrhagia–Irregular, heavy bleeding.

Oligomenorrhea–Infrequent menses. Greater than 35-day intervals.

Polymenorrhea–Menses occurring with abnormal frequency.

4

Amenorrhea

WHAT IS IT?

- Amenorrhea is the absence of menstrual bleeding. It is a symptom, not a diagnosis.
- Primary amenorrhea is the absence of spontaneous uterine bleeding and secondary sexual characteristics by age 14 or the absence of spontaneous uterine bleeding by age 16 with otherwise normal development.
- Secondary amenorrhea is a 6-month absence of menstrual bleeding in a woman with regular menses or a 12-month absence of menstrual bleeding in a woman with previous oligomenorrhea.
- Oligomenorrhea is the reduction in the frequency of menses, with an interval longer than 35 days, but less than 3 months.
- Cryptomenorrhea is hidden menstruation; menstruation occurs, but makes no external appearance because of uterine or vaginal obstruction.

ETIOLOGY

Causes of amenorrhea are multiple and include, but are not limited to, changes in the hypothalamus, pituitary gland, ovaries, uterus, adrenal glands, outlet tract, thyroid gland, and spine; systemic or chronic disease, extremes of weight and exercise, physical or mental stress, and medications; and normal physiologic processes such as pregnancy, breast-feeding, and menopause.

Hypothalamus

Alterations of the rhythmic secretions of gonadotropin-releasing hormone (GnRH) from excessive exercise, stress, or medications can cause a decrease in follicle-stimulating hormone (FSH) and luteinizing hormone (LH). The subsequent decline in estrogen and progesterone results in amenorrhea. In addition, extreme or rapid changes in weight and anorexia nervosa also influence the neuroendocrine function of the hypothalamus.

Pituitary Gland

Adenomas, prolactinomas, and other benign tumors of the pituitary gland can cause excessive production of prolactin (hyperprolactinemia), which results in amenorrhea. Other causes of hyperprolactinemia include stress, frequent or vigorous activity, nipple stimulation, and medications (including some birth control pills, ulcer medications, and psychotropic medications). Hyperprolactinemia causes amenorrhea by a negative feedback mechanism to the anterior pituitary that results in decreased production of FSH and LH.

Technical Note

- Prolactin secretion is under the influence of thyroid-releasing hormone (TRH), which is secreted by the pituitary in response to nipple stimulation. Inhibition of prolactin is controlled by prolactin-inhibiting hormone (PIH) and dopamine.
- Hypopituitary malfunction caused by conditions such as empty sella syndrome, Sheehan's syndrome (postpartum ischemic necrosis of the anterior pituitary), and Simmonds' syndrome (atrophy of the pituitary), results in decreased production of FSH and LH and subsequent amenorrhea.

Ovaries

Turner's syndrome (XO) is a genetic disorder whereby ovaries are not present at birth or are devoid of germ cells, karyotype 45 X, instead of 46 XX. The absence of ovaries implies no or minimal production of estrogen and progesterone.

In premature ovarian failure, the ovaries do not respond to pituitary hormones.

Infections, tumors, and radiation therapy all have potential impact on ovarian hormone secretion and can result in amenorrhea.

Polycystic ovary syndrome (PCOS) is a condition that manifests with increased levels of estrogen, the absence of ovulation, and minimal or no progesterone, resulting in amenorrhea.

Uterus

Intrauterine adhesions as seen in Asherman's syndrome and endometriosis disrupt the ability of the endometrium to respond appropriately to estrogen and progesterone, possibly resulting in amenorrhea.

Adrenal Glands

Causes of amenorrhea attributable to adrenal gland dysfunction include the following:
- Tumors, which frequently cause hypercortisolemia
- Cushing's syndrome (i.e., hypersecretion of the adrenal cortex)
- Administration of large doses of the adrenocortical hormones, such as prednisone

---

Technical Note

Benign tumors of the pituitary and adrenals are common, and the presence of a tumor does not imply that this is the cause of Cushing's syndrome.

Outlet Tract

Mechanical problems such as transverse vaginal septum, imperforate hymen, cervical stenosis, and agenesis affect patency from the uterus to the vaginal introitus and interfere with the outflow of menstrual blood.

Thyroid

Hypothyroidism results in increased TRH production from the pituitary. Increased TRH induces an increase in prolactin secretion, which, in turn, causes amenorrhea.

Hyperthyroidism causes amenorrhea by interfering with the production of FSH and LH.

Spinal Misalignment

Nerves of the sympathetic trunk innervate the uterus and ovaries via the hypogastric plexus. From this plexus, branches are given to the pelvic plexuses that supply the pelvic viscera. Inadequate or aberrant innervation can interfere with normal ovarian and uterine function.

Chronic or Systemic Disease

Chronic or systemic diseases such as those caused by liver or kidney dysfunction are causes of amenorrhea.

Pregnancy

Pregnancy is the most common cause of secondary amenorrhea in women of reproductive age. Once implantation occurs, the lining of the uterus, which normally sheds as menstrual blood, changes morphologically to become the decidua. The decidua ultimately becomes the placenta, which nourishes the fertilized egg and subsequently the fetus.

Extremes of Weight

Low body weight as seen with athletes, or in conditions such as anorexia nervosa or bulimia, results in diminished levels of estrogen, a decrease that predisposes to amenorrhea. In addition, estrogen is stored and synthesized in adipose tissue under the influence of the enzyme aromatase. In obesity or excessive weight there is the potential for excess estrogen, which can cause amenorrhea.

Excessive Exercise

Activities that require rigorous training, such as ballet, long-distance running, swimming, or gymnastics, may interrupt ovarian function, resulting in amenorrhea. The hormone leptin alerts the brain to the amount of fat in the body. If the percentage of body fat is too low (less than 15% to 17%), menstrual function is compromised.

Stressors

Physical, emotional, or mental stress can cause amenorrhea by interfering with the delicate neuroendocrine processes.

DIAGNOSIS

Diagnosis requires a comprehensive history, physical examination, blood analysis, and special studies where indicated.

History

See Table 4-1 for diagnostic clues in the history.

Table 4-1

Diagnostic Clues: History	
Amenorrhea with comorbid symptoms of	Is suggestive of
Depression and mood swings	Cushing's syndrome
Ease of bruising	Cushing's syndrome
Feelings of constipation	Imperforate hymen
Fever or cough	Pulmonary tuberculosis
Galactorrhea	Pituitary tumor, hyperprolactinemia
Generalized fatigue	Cushing's syndrome
Headaches	Pituitary tumor
Hirsutism	Adrenal or ovarian tumor, Cushing's syndrome
Hot flashes or night sweats	Menopause
Increase in skin pigmentation	Adrenal cortex failure
Intolerance to cold	Hypothyroidism
Intolerance to heat	Hyperthyroidism
Loss of axillary or pubic hair	Adrenal cortex or pituitary insufficiency
Loss of vision	Pituitary tumor
Low back pain	Imperforate hymen, lumbopelvic misalignments
Lower abdominal cramping	Imperforate hymen
Monthly or cyclic lower abdominal pain	Imperforate hymen
Nausea and vomiting	Pituitary tumor, pregnancy
Purple striations of the abdomen	Cushing's syndrome
Rectal pressure or cramping	Imperforate hymen
Vaginal pressure	Imperforate hymen
Weight gain	PCOS, pregnancy
Weight loss	Anorexia nervosa

Table 4-2

Diagnostic Clues: Physical Examination	
Amenorrhea with physical examination evidence of	Is suggestive of
Centripetal obesity	Cushing's syndrome
Distended abdomen	Imperforate hymen
Edema of the hands and legs	Turner's syndrome
Enlarged thyroid	Thyroid disease
Enlarged uterus	Pregnancy, imperforate hymen
Hirsutism	Cushing's syndrome, androgen excess
Hyperglycemia	Cushing's syndrome
Lactation in the absence of breast-feeding	Hyperprolactinemia, pituitary tumor
Low-set ears, widely spaced eyes	Turner's syndrome
Moon facies (rounded and red)	Cushing's syndrome
Muscle wasting	Cushing's syndrome
Osteoporosis	Menopause, Cushing's syndrome
Poor wound healing or thinning skin	Cushing's syndrome
Purple striations of the abdomen	Cushing's syndrome
Short stature	Turner's syndrome
Webbing of the neck	Turner's syndrome

Physical Examination

See Table 4-2 for diagnostic clues in the physical examination.
   Special diagnostic tests.

PELVIC EXAMINATION

A pelvic examination is performed to rule out conditions such as imperforate hymen or cervical stenosis.

Figure 4-1[*]

[*]Summarized from Zavanelli-Morgan BA: Institute of Women's Health and Integrative Medicine, Oct. 2005, and Speroff L, Fritz MA: *Clinical gynecologic endocrinology and infertility*, ed 7, Philadelphia, 2005, Lippincott Williams & Wilkins.

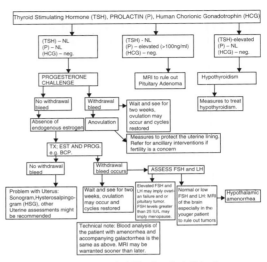

FIGURE 4-1 Amenorrhea blood analysis flow chart.

MANAGEMENT

Management is predicated on an accurate diagnosis. Select strategies include the following:

Hyperprolactinemia Without a Pituitary Tumor

- In the absence of pituitary tumor, Vitex (chaste berry) is a proven option in the management of amenorrhea caused by hyperprolactinemia. In one study, 52 women with prolactinemia who were given Vitex extract (20 mg capsule daily for 3 months) noted reduction in prolactin release, shortened luteal phases, and elimination of any defects in luteal progesterone synthesis. Dosage recommendations: 40 drops of Vitex tincture daily or 20 mg of standardized extract daily.

Pituitary tumor and hyperprolactinemia. Amenorrhea caused by a pituitary tumor or hyperprolactinemia may require specialized medical management, including the following:

- Estrogen replacement therapy. Careful monitoring of the tumor is necessary.

Table 4-3

Advanced Diagnostic Procedures	
Amenorrhea caused by	May be diagnosed by
Asherman's syndrome (intrauterine adhesions)	Hysteroscopy
Cushing's syndrome	24-hour urinary free cortisol levels greater than 50–100 mcg/day
	Dexamethasone suppression test to determine the source of the excess adrenocorticotropic hormone (ACTH)
	Corticotropin-releasing hormone (CRH) stimulation test to distinguish between pituitary adenomas, ectopic ACTH syndrome, or cortisol-secreting adrenal tumors
	Dexamethasone and CRH tests also help differentiate between Cushing's syndrome and conditions that may mimic Cushing's syndrome, such as PCOS and syndrome X; these conditions do not manifest elevated cortisol levels
	Computed tomography (CT) scan or magnetic resonance imaging (MRI) of the pituitary and adrenals to determine presence of a tumor
	Petrosal sinus sampling to differentiate between pituitary adenoma and ectopic ACTH syndrome
Pituitary tumors	MRI
Turner's syndrome	Karyotyping

- Dopamine agonists such as carbergoline, bromocriptine, or pergolide. The goal of these medications is to increase estrogen levels by reducing prolactin levels. An added bonus is that they can help to restore fertility. There is some concern about fetal malformation occurring as a result of dopamine agonists.
- Transsphenoidal surgery

Stress

Stress-induced amenorrhea requires modifications to the activities that promote stress. In addition, herbs such as chaste berry (Vitex), one capsule of the standardized extract daily, or rhodiola, 200 mg/day, may restore menses.

Polycystic Ovary Syndrome

Progesterone therapy has restored menses in women with amenorrhea caused by PCOS. Natural progesterone creams applied during the secretory phase restore bleeding in many cases of PCOS. Concurrently, obesity should be managed (see Chapter 28).

Imperforate Hymen

Amenorrhea caused by imperforate hymen is surgically corrected by a skilled gynecologist following estrogenization of the hymen and vagina to prevent scarring and potential recurrence.

Spinal Misalignment

Inadequate or aberrant innervation can interfere with normal ovarian and uterine function and can be a primary or contributing cause of amenorrhea. Correction of misalignments in the lower thoracic and lumbopelvic spines has been anecdotally reported to restore menses.

Diet and Exercise

Amenorrhea caused by excessive exercise or inadequate diet requires modifications to these activities and may necessitate collaboration with coaches, dietitians, physicians, and family members. Oral contraceptives may be used to induce bleeding and to protect against osteopenia and osteoporosis if modifications are not possible.

Clinical Pearl

Hypogonadotrophic states (i.e., prepubertal, hypothalamic dysfunction, pituitary dysfunction):
    Serum FSH less than 5 IU/L
    Serum LH less than 5 IU/L
Hypergonadotrophic states (i.e., postmenopausal, castrate, ovarian failure):
    Serum FSH greater than 20 IU/L
    Serum LH greater than 40 IU/L

5

Birth Control

Birth control methods should be considered by any woman of childbearing age who wishes to engage in sexual activity but does not desire pregnancy.

BIRTH CONTROL METHODS

- All methods come with some risk, compromise, and responsibility.
- The only foolproof, risk-free method is abstinence.
- Approximately 90% of sexually active women who do not use any contraceptive become pregnant within 1 year.

CONSIDERATIONS

- Values
- Religious beliefs and practices
- Safety
- Effectiveness
- Fertility awareness (there is typically a maximum of 7 days within the cycle when a woman can conceive)

BIRTH CONTROL CHOICES

- Natural family planning (NFP)—may be used to prevent pregnancy or to maximize the chances of conception; most NFP methods are based on a sperm life of 72 hours and an ovum life after ovulation estimated at 24 hours and up to 48 hours when ovulation occurs in both ovaries
- Hormones—combined estrogen and progesterone derivatives or progesterone derivatives administered orally, by injection, as vaginal inserts, or by intrauterine device (IUD)

- Barrier methods—cervical cap, diaphragm, spermicidal sponge, female condoms
- Insertion devices—IUD, NuvaRing, Essure
- Tubal ligation
- Hysterectomy

Natural Family Planning Methods

- **Symptothermal.** Combines the basal body temperature (BBT), the cervical mucus, and the position and texture of the cervix, which softens and rises at ovulation.
- **Billings (cervical mucus).** Following menses, cervical mucus is scant; as ovulation approaches the mucus becomes more abundant and wet, peaks in wetness at ovulation, and becomes fluid and slippery. After ovulation, the mucus becomes thicker, less slippery, and more hostile to sperm.
- **Basal body temperature.** The BBT rises immediately after ovulation as a result of rising systemic levels of progesterone. The "safe" days begin 3 days after the rise in temperature.
- **Rhythm.** The formula for calculating safe days assumes that the interval from ovulation to the onset of menses is consistently 14 days. The last safe day is calculated by subtracting 18 from the length of the cycle, and the first safe day is calculated by subtracting 11 from the length of the cycle. For example, a woman with a 29-day cycle has a last safe day at day 11 (29 − 18) and a first late safe day at day 18 (29 − 11). In the event that intercourse occurs on day 11, by day 14 sperm is nonviable. Ovulation occurs on day 15; within 48 hours the egg is nonviable, and intercourse can resume on day 18. This method assumes regular cycle intervals and ovulation from one ovary or simultaneous ovulation from both ovaries.

Advantages
- Safe and inexpensive
- Mutual responsibility is encouraged
- No barriers to interrupt lovemaking
- No chemicals or hormones to interfere with the body's natural milieu

Disadvantages
- Some women do not have recognizable cervical mucus or BBT patterns

- Too bothersome
- Several months of records and charts are needed

Use effectiveness

- From 53% to 99%, with an average of 85% based on compliance

Hormonal Methods

Combination estrogen and progesterone

- Oral contraceptive
- Ortho Evra patch
- NuvaRing
- Emergency contraception

Progesterone only

- Depo-Provera injection
- Minipill
- Insertion capsules (Norplant has been taken off the market, and Implanon is awaiting U.S. Food and Drug Administration [FDA] approval)
- Progestasert IUD
- Emergency contraception

Combination methods. The combined estrogen and progesterone birth control methods work by maintaining systemic levels of estrogen that blunt the triggering of the hypothalamic secretions of gonadotropin-releasing hormone (GnRH) factors specific to follicle-stimulating hormone (FSH) and luteinizing hormone (LH) secretion. Estrogen simultaneously inhibits FSH production and decreases follicle development, thereby limiting ovulation. The progestins inhibit LH release, interfering with ovulation. The cervical mucus, under the influence of progesterone, becomes thick and hostile to sperm, and the fallopian tubes have decreased motility.

Combination oral contraception. The combined birth control pill contains both progestins and estrogen; 28-day and 21-day packs are available. Both contain 21 days of pills with hormones; 28-day packs also contain seven inactive pills. Menstruation occurs during the fourth week. The birth control pill Seasonale has 11 weeks of oral contraceptives with 1 week of inactive pills for four menses per year.

- Action: inhibits ovulation and thickens cervical mucus
- Theoretic effectiveness: 99%
- Use effectiveness: 95% to 99%

Advantages

- Convenient and effective; does not interfere with sexual spontaneity
- Decreased menstrual blood loss and menorrhagia
- Reduced incidence of endometrial cancer
- Reduced incidence of ovarian cysts and ovarian cancer

Disadvantages and side effects

- Thrombophlebitis
- Deep vein thrombosis
- Hypertension
- Pulmonary embolism
- Breast tenderness
- Headaches, migraine, irritability
- Depression
- Weight gain or loss
- Decreased libido
- Offers no protection against sexually transmitted diseases (STDs), human immunodeficiency virus (HIV), or hepatitis virus

Complications and contraindications

- Liver disease or abnormal liver function tests
- Inflammation of the optic nerve/double vision
- Smokers over age 35
- Hypertension
- Diabetes
- Active cholecystitis
- Hypercholesterolemia
- Antiseizure medications
- Altered vitamin and mineral metabolism

Technical Note

The birth control pill Yasmin contains the progestin drospirenone, which may increase potassium levels and cause heart disease. In addition, individuals with a history of adrenal, kidney, or liver disease should not take Yasmin. Yasmin is a combination pill containing ethinyl estradiol and drospirenone, a progestin derived from spironolactone, unlike most other birth control progestins, which are derived from testosterone. Yasmin works as an antiandrogen and is an effective aid in the resolution of acne and hirsutism. Side effects of Yasmin include headache, menstrual changes, breast tenderness, abdominal cramps, bloating, nausea, and vaginal discharge.

Progestin-only Oral Contraception

Minipill. This is an oral tablet taken daily that contains progestins only. It is available in 28-day packs in which all the pills are active. Menstruation (when present) occurs during the fourth week.

- Action: thickens cervical mucus and may inhibit ovulation
- Theoretic effectiveness: 97%
- Use effectiveness: approximately 92% to 97%

Advantages

- Minimal maintenance
- Useful for women who should not use estrogen

Disadvantages and side effects

- Breakthrough bleeding
- Depression
- Acne
- Headaches
- Must be taken at the same time every day with no more than a 3-hour delay or it may be rendered ineffective; a backup method then would be required for the remainder of the pack

Complications and contraindications. Although this is a progestin-only pill, complications and contraindications are reported to be the same as those of combined oral contraceptive pills (OCPs) and include the following:

- History of liver disease
- Meningioma
- History of thrombophlebitis or thrombosis

Ortho Evra patch. This is a square patch containing the hormones ethinyl estradiol and norelgestromin. The patch is replaced once a week for 3 weeks. The absence of a patch during the fourth week prompts withdrawal bleeding. The patch can be placed on the buttocks, stomach, upper torso, or upper outer arm.

- Action: inhibits ovulation and thickens cervical mucus
- Theoretic effectiveness: 97% to 99%
- Use effectiveness: 95% to 99%

Each patch remains effective for up to 9 days but ideally should be replaced once a week on the same day. The patch may be less effective for women who weigh more than 198 pounds.

Medications and herbs that may impair effectiveness include the following:

- Some oral antifungal agents
- The antibiotic rifampin
- Some anti-HIV protease inhibitors
- Certain antiseizure medications
- The herb St. John's wort

Advantages

- Pregnancy protection for 1 month without the need to take a daily pill
- Does not interfere with sexual spontaneity
- May predispose to lighter, shorter periods
- Fertility returns once use is terminated

Disadvantages and side effects

- Skin reaction at the site
- Menstrual cramps
- Alterations in vision
- Affords no protection against STDs
- Intermenstrual spotting or bleeding
- Mood swings
- Depression
- Breast tenderness
- Alterations of weight
- Headaches
- Nausea
- Amenorrhea
- Menorrhagia

Complications and contraindications

- Pregnancy
- Menorrhagia
- Thrombophlebitis or thromboembolic disorders
- Impaired liver function
- Smoker over age 35
- Heart disease or stroke

- Uncontrolled high blood pressure
- Known or suspected estrogen-dependent neoplasias

NuvaRing. Theoretically, this device has the same side effects and contraindications as the combined OCPs because it contains both estrogen and progestin.

The NuvaRing is a flexible circular device that is inserted into the vagina once every month. It releases hormones (ethinyl estradiol and etonogestrel) for 3 weeks and is removed in the fourth week, prompting withdrawal bleeding.

- Action: inhibits ovulation and thickens cervical mucus
- Theoretic effectiveness: 99%
- Use effectiveness: 95% to 99%
  Factors that impair use effectiveness include the following:
- Unopened packages exposed to very high temperatures or direct sunlight
- The ring slips out of the vagina and is not expediently replaced
- The ring is kept in the vagina for more than 3 weeks or is not kept in the vagina for 3 consecutive weeks

Advantages
- Pregnancy protection for 1 month with minimal maintenance
- Steady release of hormones
- Does not interfere with sexual spontaneity
- Regular and lighter menstrual periods
- Once terminated, fertility is rapidly restored

Disadvantages and side effects
- May increase vaginal discharge, vaginal irritation, and vaginal infection
- May cause unscheduled bleeding
- Breast tenderness
- Mood swings
- Depression
- Nausea

Complications and contraindications
- Pregnancy
- Menorrhagia
- Thrombophlebitis or thromboembolic disorders
- Impaired liver function
- Smoker over age 35
- Heart disease or stroke

- Uncontrolled high blood pressure
- Known or suspected estrogen-dependent neoplasias

Barrier Methods

- Cervical cap
- Diaphragm
- Contraceptive sponge
- Male and female condoms

Advantages

- High rate of reliability
- Decrease the incidence of cervical cancer
- Afford some protection against STDs

Disadvantages

- May interfere with sexual spontaneity
- Allergic reaction to the latex
- Recurrent cystitis or candidiasis
- The cap and diaphragm require reapplication of contraceptive jelly between acts of intercourse
- Can be messy

Effectiveness

- Diaphragm: approximately 80% (80% to 94%)
- Cervical cap without having birthed children: 80% to 90%
- Cervical cap with vaginal birth: approximately 60% to 80%
- Contraceptive sponge: approximately 80% (71% to 97%)
- Condoms: approximately 90% (64% to 97%)

Insertion Devices

Intrauterine device. The intrauterine device (IUD) is the most popular reversible method worldwide; however, in the United States it is currently used by only 1% of the population. It is a T-shaped plastic device that may be coiled with copper or coated with progestin derivatives (Figure 5-1).

- Action: irritates the uterine lining, impairs sperm motility, interferes with fertilization, and inhibits implantation. Some brands release low levels of progesterone, which thickens cervical mucus, further inhibiting sperm motility. In addition, the progestins may impair fertilization.
  - The Paragard Copper T IUD, once inserted, can provide protection for up to 10 years.

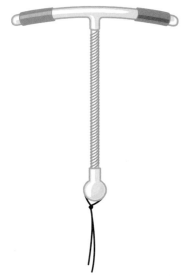

FIGURE 5-1 An example of an IUD. (From Hacker NF, Moore JG, Gambone JC: *Essentials of obstetrics and gynecology,* ed 4, Philadelphia, 2004, WB Saunders.)

- The Mirena IUD, once inserted, can provide protection for up to 5 years. Releases progestins.
- The Progestasert IUD, once inserted, can provide protection for up to 1 year. Releases progestins.
- Theoretic effectiveness is 99%.
- Use effectiveness is 94% to 99%.

   The IUD is ideally suited for parous females in a monogamous relationship.

Advantages
- Provides long-term birth control with minimal maintenance
- Does not interfere with sexual spontaneity
- Absence of the systemic side effects that can occur with oral hormonal birth control methods

Disadvantages and side effects
- Dysmenorrhea
- Spotting between periods
- Paragard IUD may increase menorrhagia
- Some women experience low back pain

- Increased vaginal discharge
- Does not provide protection against STDs, HIV, or hepatitis B

Complications and contraindications

- There may be an increased risk for pelvic inflammatory disease (PID), especially during the first 3 weeks following insertion and in a woman with multiple partners.
- The IUD may perforate through the wall of the uterus at the time of insertion.
- There is an approximately 10% expulsion rate within the first year, typically caused by the method of insertion or insertion in a nonparous woman.
- Rarely, pregnancy may occur with an IUD in place. In the event of a pregnancy, most authorities recommend removal of the IUD. Pregnancy with an IUD in place may also cause sepsis, septic abortion, and maternal death.

EMERGENCY CONTRACEPTION

Contraceptive Pills

Combined oral contraceptives (ethinyl estradiol and norgestrel or levonorgestrel)

- Administered in two doses, the first within 72 hours of unprotected intercourse and the second exactly 12 hours later or both pills taken at the same time
- Approximately 75% to 80% effective

Oral contraceptives containing levonorgestrel alone (Plan B)

- Administered in two doses, the first within 72 hours of unprotected intercourse and the second exactly 12 hours later or both pills taken at the same time
- Approximately 89% effective

Clinical Pearl

Emergency contraceptive pills are often called "the morning after pill." This is a misnomer because they do not have to be taken the morning after. Some work for up to 5 days, and they are never taken as only one pill.

Copper-containing IUD

- Insertion within 5 days of unprotected intercourse
- Approximately 99% effective
- Difficult to find physicians who will insert

Mifepristone (RU 486)
- Given through the seventh week of pregnancy
- Also called "the abortion pill"

Norplant/Implanon

Norplant is a system of six slow-release levonorgestrel capsules implanted into the upper arm. It was taken off the market because of problems with insertion, removal, localized infection, and scarring. The updated single-capsule version, Implanon, is currently awaiting approval by the FDA. It is being used with success in other countries.

6

Bladder Pain Syndrome (Interstitial Cystitis)

WHAT IS IT?

Bladder pain syndrome is a chronic condition of unknown etiology marked by irritation/inflammation of the lining of the bladder wall.

WHO GETS IT?

Bladder pain syndrome occurs almost exclusively in women.

ETIOLOGY

The cause of bladder pain syndrome is unknown. Proposed causes include the following:
- Autoimmune response following an acute bladder infection
- Allergic reaction to urinary substrates
- Irritation to the nerves of the sacral plexus

SIGNS AND SYMPTOMS

- Urinary frequency
- Urinary urgency
- Pain in the bladder ranging in intensity from mild pressure to severe pain
- Pain in the lower abdomen and pelvis
- Sensation of increased pressure in the lower abdomen
- Dyspareunia
- Dysmenorrhea

DIAGNOSIS

- Rule out conditions such as urinary tract infections (UTIs), sexually transmitted diseases (STDs), reproductive tract malignancy, and endometriosis
- Signs and symptoms listed above
- Urinalysis
- STD screening
- Pelvic examination
- Definitive diagnosis is by cystoscopy, which is used to detect signs of inflammation, bleeding, bladder capacity, and bladder wall flexibility

MANAGEMENT

- Self-help:
  - Evaluate the diet for factors that increase the sensation of frequency and urgency; suspected triggers include dairy, caffeine, high-acid foods, and artificial sweeteners
- Physical therapy:
  - Biofeedback for bladder training, pain control, and muscle relaxation
  - Transcutaneous electrical nerve stimulation (TENS) for pain modification
  - Spinal manipulation with emphasis directed at the sacral nerves
- Medications:
  - Elmiron, nonsteroidal antiinflammatory drugs (NSAIDs), pain medications, and antidepressants
- Procedures:
  - Bladder instillation
  - Sacral nerve stimulation implants (see Appendix)

7

Breast Conditions

BREAST CANCER
What Is It?
Breast cancer is a malignant neoplasm of the breast that is classified as *in situ* if contained or *invasive* if it has infiltrated the surrounding tissue.

Types of Breast Cancer
There are several types of breast cancer, with the majority falling into two categories: ductal carcinoma, which begins in the epithelial cells lining the ducts, and lobular carcinoma, which begins in the milk-secreting glands of the breasts. Breast cancer also can arise from adipose tissue, connective tissue, and the skin.

Ductal carcinoma is the most common of all breast cancers, and ductal carcinoma in situ has the highest cure rate of all the cancers.

Ductal carcinoma is further subdivided by growth patterns, which are micropapillary, cribriform, solid, or comedo. The comedo growth pattern is considered the most aggressive.

Breast cancer is now the leading cause of death in women ages 35 to 54 and the second leading cause of cancer death in women of all ages. Currently one in eight women in the United States will be diagnosed with breast cancer. The majority of breast cancers occur in women over 50.

Who Gets It?
Women of all ages get breast cancer, although most cases occur in women over 40 and 75% occur in women over 50. According

to the National Cancer Institute (NCI), the incidence of breast cancer for different age categories is as follows:

- Ages 20 to 30 years: 1 in 2000
- Ages 30 to 40 years: 1 in 250
- Ages 40 to 50 years: 1 in 67
- Ages 50 to 60 years: 1 in 35
- Ages 60 to 70 years: 1 in 28
- Lifetime: 1 in 8

Etiology and Risk Factors

- Personal history of breast cancer. Women who have had breast cancer in one breast are more likely to redevelop breast cancer.
- Family history. Approximately 20% of women with breast cancer have a family history of breast cancer. The primary breast cancer gene is autosomal dominant, maternal linkage.
- Overweight/obesity. The enzyme aromatase is present in adipose tissue; common sites for aromatase include the lateral breasts. Aromatase facilitates the conversion of the estrogen derivative estrone to the more potent estradiol. Excessive levels of estradiol can predispose to breast cancer.
- Hormonal influences. High or sustained levels of estrogens increase the rate of growth of all cells, including the genetically damaged cells that can cause cancer.
- Nulliparity and not carrying children to term.
- Long reproductive life (early onset of menarche, i.e., before age 12; or late menopause, i.e., after age 55).
- Delaying pregnancy (having a first full-term pregnancy after age 30).
- Exogenous estrogen use, including estrogen replacement therapy (ERT) and high-estrogen birth control pills.
- Dietary factors. Eating foods that have been treated with hormones may increase the overall estrogen load, which can predispose to breast cancer.
- Xenoestrogens. Estrogen "look-alikes" found in pesticides, plastics, and other environmental sources bind to estrogen receptor sites with seemingly deleterious consequences.
- Breast cancer genes (BRCA1 and BRCA2). There is increasing evidence to suggest that breast cancer is caused by the growth of genetically damaged cells that gradually accumulate in the

body over time. Approximately 1 in 400 U.S. women carry a germ-line mutation for the breast cancer gene BRCA1. BRCA1 and BRCA2 carriers have a 50% to 85% lifetime risk of breast cancer, ovarian cancer, or both. BRCA2 carriers appear to have a higher risk of male breast cancer, which accounts for only 1% of all breast cancers.

- Several other genes have been identified that also may increase breast cancer risk. These include Noey 2, a genetic defect inherited from the father; BRCA3; BARD 1; and p53, all of which appear to play a role in increasing breast cancer risk.
- Repeated chest radiation, as occurs in conditions such as Hodgkin's disease.

Signs and Symptoms

- Often there are no outward signs of breast cancer.
- When signs occur, they can include the following:
  - A firm but not rock-hard mass or lump in one of the breasts, often in the upper or lower outer quadrants. The mass may have irregular borders and typically is not moveable.
  - A thickening or "orange peel" appearance of the breast.
  - Dilated or aggressive venous patterns on the breast.
  - A mass in the area of the armpit.
  - A depression or bulge in the skin of the breast.
  - Nipple discharge, which often is bloody.
  - Changes in the nipple, including change in nipple direction or retraction of the nipple, or changes in nipple sensation.
  - A nonhealing sore on the breast or nipple.
  - Swelling in the arm or hand.
  - Back (bone) pain.

Screening and Diagnosis

- Breast examinations. Monthly breast self-examinations and expert clinician breast examinations are critical in the early identification of a breast lump.
- Mammography (x-ray of the breast) can be useful in identifying and locating the lump. The procedure involves exposing the breasts to small amounts of radiation.
- Fine-needle biopsy to assess the fluids in the mass.
- Excisional biopsy to remove the lump and assess the tissues.

- Laboratory analysis, including complete blood count (CBC) and liver function tests.
- Chest x-ray.
- Ultrasound can identify masses missed by mammography and differentially diagnose a solid mass from a fluid-filled mass.
- Pathologic review of biopsy, and estrogen and progesterone receptor determination and S-phase determination.
- Bone scan should be performed if symptoms suggest bony metastasis, if alkaline phosphatase is elevated, or if widespread disease is suspected.
- Ductal lavage is used to identify cancerous and precancerous cells in the milk ducts of the breast. The procedure involves injecting saline solution into fluid-producing ducts. The saline solution then is suctioned out along with cells from the epithelial lining of the ductal system. The fluid is analyzed for normal, atypical, or malignant cells.
- Thermography. Breast thermography can be used to evaluate the degree of vascular dilation of the breasts. This measure is compared with the degree of dilation during lactation when estrogen levels are elevated. Prolonged exposure to estrogen is a risk factor for breast cancer. The degree of vascular dilation in the breast may provide an assessment of the levels of estrogen in the breast.

    There is evidence to suggest that the breasts can hold 10 to 50 times more estrogen than identified on a typical blood test. Excess estrogen stimulates breast tissue and dilates blood vessels. Dilated blood vessels are more visible on thermograms than nondilated vessels because they have more blood and heat flowing through them.

Management

Breast cancer prevention strategies
Lifestyle factors
- Maintain recommended body weight
- Breast-feed
- Have children before age 30
- Exercise (e.g., a daily walking program)
- Avoid drinking water from plastic bottles that have been sitting in hot temperatures, such as in a hot car on a summer day
- Reduce alcohol consumption

Diet

- The diet should be rich in cruciferous vegetables and other sources of indole 3-carbinol, which has been demonstrated to shunt the liver's metabolism of estrogen to the 2-hydroxy (2-OH) estrogen derivative, which is less potent and may have protective effects against breast cancer.
- Sources of indole 3-carbinol include the cruciferous vegetables, broccoli, kale, cauliflower, cabbage, brussels sprouts, collard greens, and bok choy.
- Phytoestrogens such as soy and red clover have molecular structures that resemble estrogen. Diets containing phytoestrogens may promote overall hormonal health and aid in the elimination of xenoestrogens. Red clover can be used to stabilize hormonal fluctuations.
- Lignans. Diets overloaded with refined foods are often deficient in lignans. Studies in Finland have shown that women with blood levels of enterolactone above 34 nmol/L had marked reduction in risk for breast cancers. Once ingested, lignans are converted by the intestinal microflora to enterolactone and enterodiol, which are mammalian lignans.
- Supplementation with standardized lignans may decrease the risk of breast cancer.
- Green tea catechins.
- Lycopene (tomatoes, red peppers, pink grapefruit).
- Modify exposure to xenoestrogens and other exogenous estrogens.
- Use glass containers for storage instead of plastic.
- Drink pure filtered water.
- Eat meats, poultry, and dairy products from nonhormonally fattened cattle.
- To minimize contamination by pesticides, eat organic vegetables.
- Avoid or minimize the use of high-estrogen medications or birth control methods.

Nutritional supplementation

- Calcium D-glucarate to aid in the elimination of xenoestrogens and enhance the function of the intestinal flora by combating the action of the bacteria with beta-glucuronidase activity.
- Coenzyme Q_{10} 300 mg/day
- Selenium 67 mcg/day
- Vitamin C 5000 mg/day

- Vitamin E 400 to 1000 IU/day
- Vitamin A less than 5000 IU/day
- Folate (5-methyltetrahydrofolate)
- Vitamin B$_6$ 50 to 100 mg/day

Screening
- Breast examinations
  - Breast self-examinations performed monthly
  - Clinician-performed breast examinations yearly after age 20

   The American Cancer Society recommends that a baseline mammogram be performed between ages 35 and 40 and recommends yearly mammography for all women 40 and older.

   The NCI recommends mammogram screening every 1 to 2 years for all women 40 and older and sooner for women with a family history of breast cancer. Annual mammograms are recommended beginning 10 years earlier than the age at which the relative was diagnosed.

Clinical Pearl

Mammography remains an effective tool for the early detection of breast cancer in women over 50. In younger women, there is an increased likelihood of false-positive results because of increased density of the breast tissue. Thermography, magnetic resonance imaging (MRI), ultrasound, and ductal lavage may be better screening tools. Breast self-examination continues to be effective in women who find a breast mass before their annual mammogram.

Stages of breast cancer (from the American Joint Committee on Cancer)

- **Stage 0.** In situ ("in place") disease in which the cancerous cells are in their original location within normal breast tissue. Known as either ductal carcinoma in situ (DCIS) or lobular carcinoma in situ (LCIS), depending on the type of cells involved and the location. This is a precancerous condition, and only a small percentage of DCIS tumors progress to become invasive cancers. There is some controversy within the medical community on how best to treat DCIS.

- **Stage I.** Tumor less than 2 cm in diameter with no spread beyond the breast.
- **Stage IIA.** Tumor 2 to 5 cm in size without spread to axillary (armpit) lymph nodes or tumor less than 2 cm in size with spread to axillary lymph nodes.
- **Stage IIB.** Tumor greater than 5 cm in size without spread to axillary lymph nodes or tumor 2 to 5 cm in size with spread to axillary lymph nodes.
- **Stage IIIA.** Tumor smaller than 5 cm in size with spread to axillary lymph nodes, which are attached to each other or to other structures, or tumor larger than 5 cm in size with spread to axillary lymph nodes.
- **Stage IIIB.** The tumor has penetrated outside the breast to the skin of the breast or the chest wall or has spread to lymph nodes inside the chest wall along the sternum.
- **Stage IV.** A tumor of any size with spread beyond the region of the breast and chest wall, such as to liver, bone, or lungs.

Medical Management

Management of breast cancer depends on the type and severity of the breast cancer and can include one or more of the following: mastectomy, lumpectomy, chemotherapy, radiation, and lymph node resection (Table 7-1). In addition, breast cancer management depends on the patient's personal and family history, risk factors, the appearance of the cancer, whether the cancer cells respond to hormones, and the presence or absence of genes known to cause breast cancer.

- Mastectomy. The various forms of mastectomy are all performed under general anesthesia.
  - Subcutaneous mastectomy involves the removal of the entire breast with the exception of the nipple and areola.
  - Simple mastectomy involves removal of the entire breast, including the nipple and areola, while leaving the axillary or central lymph nodes (those in the armpit and under the arm) intact.
  - Modified radical mastectomy involves removal of the entire breast, including the nipple and areola, and an axillary dissection, which involves removal of the majority of the lymph nodes in the area.

- Radical mastectomy involves removal of the entire breast and the major muscles of the chest wall. This is an outdated procedure that nevertheless is occasionally performed.
- Lumpectomy. Local anesthesia with or without sedatives is used. An incision is made, and the lump and immediately surrounding tissues are removed and evaluated.
- Radiation therapy is directed at the tumor, the breast, the chest wall, or other tissues known or suspected to have remaining cancer cells.
- Chemotherapy may be used to help eliminate the remaining cancer cells in the breast or other parts of the body.
- Hormonal therapies in the form of drugs such as tamoxifen (Nolvadex) and raloxifene (Evista) are used to block the effects of estrogen on breast tissue.

Table 7-1

Treatment Considerations in Breast Cancer	
Stage	Treatment considerations
0	Mastectomy or lumpectomy plus radiation is the standard treatment. However, there is some controversy on how best to treat DCIS.
I	Lumpectomy (plus radiation) or mastectomy with at least "sentinel node" lymph node removal is standard treatment. Chemotherapy, hormone therapy, or both may be recommended following surgery. The presence of breast cancer in the axillary lymph nodes is useful for staging and the appropriate follow-up treatment.
II	Lumpectomy with radiation or mastectomy with axillary dissection (including the removal of the sentinel node). In addition, chemotherapy or other hormonal therapy may be recommended following surgery.
III	Mastectomy followed by chemotherapy and frequently hormonal therapy or radiation therapy.
IV	Mastectomy, radiation, chemotherapy, hormonal therapy, or some combination.

Prognosis

Five-year survival rates for individuals with breast cancer who receive appropriate treatment are as follows:

Stage	5-Year relative survival rate
0	100%
I	100%
IIA	92%
IIB	81%
IIIA	67%
IIIB	54%
IV	20%

Source: American Cancer Society Web site
www.seer.cancer.gov (last accessed May 18, 2006).

The axillary lymph nodes are the main passageway that breast cancer cells use to reach the rest of the body. Their involvement at any time strongly affects the prognosis.

Preventive mastectomy (the surgical removal of one or both breasts) is an option for women who are at very high risk for breast cancer. Possible candidates for this procedure are women who have already had one breast removed because of cancer, women with a strong family history of breast cancer, women who have a mutation in gene p53or gene BRCA1, and those who have gene BRCA2.

LYMPHEDEMA

What Is It?

Lymphedema, a common complication of procedures to treat breast cancer, is swelling of the arm caused by accumulation of lymph fluid in the soft tissues of the arm (Figure 7-1).

Who Gets It?

Between 5% and 25% of women develop lymphedema following treatment for breast cancer, including lumpectomy, mastectomy, lymph node dissection, radiation therapy, and chemotherapy.

Etiology

Breast cancer treatment frequently involves removal of portions of the axillary and surrounding lymph nodes and channels, thereby compromising the lymphatic system. In addition, the compromised immune state following many breast cancer

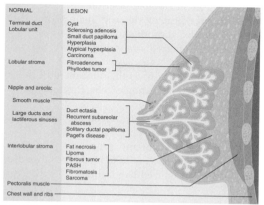

NORMAL	LESION
Terminal duct Lobular unit	Cyst Sclerosing adenosis Small duct papilloma Hyperplasia Atypical hyperplasia Carcinoma
Lobular stroma	Fibroadenoma Phyllodes tumor
Nipple and areola: Smooth muscle	
Large ducts and lactiferous sinuses	Duct ectasia Recurrent subareolar abscess Solitary ductal papilloma Paget's disease
Interlobular stroma	Fat necrosis Lipoma Fibrous tumor PASH Fibromatosis Sarcoma
Pectoralis muscle	
Chest wall and ribs	

FIGURE 7-1 Normal breast anatomy and anatomic locations of common breast lesions. (From Kumar V, Cotran R, Robbins S: *Robbins and Cotran pathologic basis of disease,* ed 7, Philadelphia, 2005, WB Saunders.)

treatments increases the chances of infection. Infection increases blood flow and hence lymphatic flow to the arm. These factors combine to cause fluid backup into the surrounding tissues and swelling.

Risk Factors

Additional risk factors for lymphedema include smoking, history of diabetes, obesity, previous surgeries to the arm, weight gain, trauma to the arm, and heat.

Signs and Symptoms

- Swelling of the arm
- Fatigue of the arm
- Sense of heaviness in the arm
- Symptoms lasting days to months

Management

- Self-help
  - Maintain diligent skin care

- Rest the arm in an elevated position
- Avoid excessive heat to the arm such as hot packs, hot weather, hot tubs, and hot showers
- Avoid using the affected arm to carry heavy objects, including shoulder bags
- Avoid clothing that restricts the movement of the arm
- Avoid blood pressure testing on the affected arm
- Avoid alcohol, smoking
- Avoid all strenuous activity, including household duties such as vacuuming
- Ensure early treatment of any infection
- Exercise (e.g., swimming, mild to moderate range-of-motion exercises with customized bandaging)

Therapeutic Aids

- Compression sleeves
- Compression bandages
- Pneumatic pumps
- Sequential gradient pumps

Physical Therapy

Complex decongestive physiotherapy followed by compression bandages. This technique involves gentle, circular, stimulating massage of the skin and lymphatic channels in the direction of the shoulder. Complex decongestive physiotherapy is applied several times a week for several weeks and should be performed by a trained therapist.

Medications

Administer diuretics along with antibiotics if infection or cellulitis is suspected.

FIBROADENOMA

What Is It?

Fibroadenoma is a benign tumor of the breast composed of fibrous and glandular tissue (Figure 7-1).

Who Gets It?

Women during their menstruating years, and more commonly younger women ages 18 to 35. Fibroadenoma is the most common breast tumor seen in adolescent girls.

Etiology

Unknown. Proposed causes include the following:
- Increased focal sensitivity to estrogen
- High-fat diets

Signs and Symptoms

- Round, rubbery, freely moveable tumor
- Nontender
- Not attached to the skin
- Clearly delineated from the surrounding tissue

Diagnosis

- By signs and symptoms
- Needle biopsy
- Mammography
- Ultrasound

Management

- Self-help
  - Monthly breast self-examinations to watch for any changes in the lump
  - Decrease in dietary fats

  Once fibroadenoma is confirmed, a wait-and-see approach may be recommended, to avoid scarring the breasts with removal.

Medications

Birth control pills to decrease associated symptoms

Procedures

- Surgical excision

FIBROCYSTIC BREAST CHANGES

What Is It?

Fibrocystic breast changes, alternatively called *fibrocystic breast disease* or *cyclic mastalgia,* is an exaggeration of the response of breast tissue to changing hormone levels. It is the most common benign condition of the breasts, occurring in as many as half of all American women.

Who Gets It?

Females during their menstruating years. Most commonly occurs in women ages 25 to 40.

Etiology

The absolute cause of fibrocystic breast changes is undetermined. Proposed causes include the following:

- Tissue response—an exaggeration of the normal response of the breasts to the fluctuating hormones.
- Hereditary—there is some evidence of familial occurrence of fibrocystic breast changes.
- Diet—dietary modifications have been shown to positively affect some of the symptoms associated with fibrocystic breasts.
- Hormones—there is some evidence that higher than normal estrogen levels or alterations in the estrogen-to-progesterone ratio can predispose to fibrocystic breast changes.
- Alterations in muscle tone, particularly within the pectoralis muscle, may affect lymphatic drainage mechanisms in the chest wall. This can lead to congestion in the tissues, which may predispose to fibrocystic breast changes.
- Postural and lifestyle habits—rounded shoulders, bad posture, and underwire bras are all factors that have the potential to interfere with normal lymphatic drainage mechanisms, thereby predisposing to fibrocystic breast changes.

Signs and Symptoms

- Lumpy breasts
- Breast pain and tenderness
- Swelling of the breast

- One or more soft, moveable lumps in either or both breasts
- Feeling of fullness in the breasts
- Nipple "zingers" or itching
- Symptoms progressively worsen after ovulation and improve after menses
- Most common sites are in the lateral quadrants of the breasts

Diagnosis

- Women who regularly perform breast self-examinations may note changes in the breasts during the cycle. The breasts become more lumpy and tender before menses and less lumpy and less tender after menses.
- Physician-administered breast examinations may reveal moveable, nonadhered, cystlike masses with clearly delineated borders in the breasts.
- Fine-needle aspiration of the cyst can be used to both diagnose and treat fibrocystic changes.
- Mammography may be used to differentially diagnose fibrocystic changes from breast cancer and other breast disorders.
- Excisional biopsy of the tissue is used to differentially diagnose fibrocystic changes from breast cancer and other breast disorders.

Management

- Self-help
  - Good breast support, such as wearing a well-made supportive bra, can provide symptom relief.
  - Regular breast self-examinations should be performed.

Dietary management

- Caffeine intake should be restricted or eliminated.
- Trans fats should be avoided.
- Excess salt should be avoided.
- Consumption of fruits and vegetables should be increased.
- Diet should include sources of omega-3 fatty acids such as flaxseed.
- Phytoestrogens such as soy (tofu and tempeh) and red clover should be introduced into the diet.
- Meats and poultry that have been hormonally treated should be avoided.

Supplementation
- Chaste berry extract 20 mg up to three times daily.
- Fish oils eicosapentaenoic acid and docosahexaenoic acid (EPA/DHA 400 to 800 mg daily. (Note: There is contradictory evidence about the efficacy of fish oils as a primary treament for fibrocystic breast changes.)
- Vitamin B_6 in a B_6 complex, up to 100 mg daily for 3 months.
- Magnesium 400 mg/day.
- Vitamin E 200 IU three times per day, beta-carotene up to 50,000 IU daily, and coenzyme Q_{10} 100 mg/day are beneficial for their antioxidant properties.

Exercise
- A good walking program, being mindful of posture
- Pectoralis stretch and strengthening exercises

Spinal manipulation
- Assessment and manipulation of the spinal areas that provide innervation to the breasts and ovaries

Massage therapy
- The muscles of the shoulder and pectoral girdle should be assessed and managed for hypertonicity and trigger points.

Modalities
- Heat modalities may be beneficial

Medications
- Low-estrogen oral contraceptives
- Bromocriptine
- Synthetic androgens

Procedures
- Needle biopsy and aspiration are concurrently diagnostic and curative.

MASTITIS

What Is It?

Inflammation/infection of the breasts.

Who Gets It?

Women who are breast-feeding. If mastitis occurs in non–breast-feeding women, it may be an indication of breast cancer.

Etiology

- Improper drainage of the milk duct, leading to inflammation
- Bacteria may enter through a crack in the nipple

Signs and Symptoms

- An area of redness (triangular flush) on the underside of the breast
- Swelling of the breast
- Pain and tenderness in the breast
- Sensation of heat on the breast
- Mild to moderate fever
- Flulike symptoms

Diagnosis

- History of breast-feeding
- Presenting symptoms
- Needle aspiration or biopsy, especially in non–breast-feeding women
- Mammography in non–breast-feeding women

Management and Prevention

- The infant should be nursed on demand.
- Adequate rest. Mastitis often is an indication that the mother is doing too much.
- Frequent nursing to unplug the duct and to keep the breasts from becoming engorged. The affected side should be nursed first and the feeding position altered to allow the breast to hang freely.
- Fit of the bra. The pressure on the tissues from a snugly fitting bra may restrict flow and predispose to inflammation. The bra should accommodate the changes in breast size.
- Feeding schedule. Missed or shortened feedings predispose to engorged and inflamed breasts.
- Position of the baby. The infant should be positioned in a manner that enables the infant to suckle effectively.
- Hot packs can be placed on the breast, and the breast massaged toward the nipple from behind the site of inflammation.

The breast should be pumped or the baby breast-fed immediately after treating the area. Hot packs increase circulation and accelerate healing and may be used with a comfrey compress. Treatment with hot packs should be follwed with ice packs to decrease inflammation.

- Cold cabbage leaves to decrease inflammation.
- The mother should drink plenty of fluids, ensure good nutrition, and supplement with a multivitamin.
- Relaxed, unhurried, thorough nursing is mandatory, with care taken to ensure cleanliness around the nipple.
- The infant should be encouraged to suckle from both breasts uniformly.
- The infant should be assessed for its ability to suckle effectively. This may necessitate alterations in the infant's feeding position, careful trigger point therapy to the muscles of the infant's jaw, and gentle manipulation of the infant's cervical spine.

Clinical Pearl

Cold cabbage leaves have been used to decrease milk supply in women who wish to discontinue breast-feeding. Weaning increases the risk of developing a breast abscess that will require surgical drainage.

Nutritional Recommendations

- Thymus support
- Sage tea in small quantities for engorgement
- Lecithin
- Green tea

The woman should inform her pediatrician of any herbal supplements she is taking while breast-feeding.

Technical Note

Although it is an effective treatment for cyclic mastalgia, chaste berry (Vitex) is not an appropriate treatment for mastitis. Its prolactin-lowering abilities are contraindicated in the nursing mother.

Spinal Manipulation

- The infant's cervical spine should be evaluated for upper cervical subluxation or torticollis, especially if the infant is favoring one breast.
- The mother's thoracic spine and cervicothoracic spine should be evaluated and adjusted as necessary.

Physical Therapy

- Ultrasound may be used.

Soft Tissue Techniques

Infant. The muscles surrounding the temporomandibular joint (TMJ), including the temporalis and the masseter, should be assessed for hypertonicity and trigger points. The pterygoids also may warrant assessment. Removing these aberrant influences may help ensure that the infant is able to latch on and suckle appropriately. Infants delivered by forceps may be predisposed to irritation in the muscles surrounding the TMJ.
Mother. Implementation of massage therapies to the muscles of the shoulder girdle and cervical and thoracic spines may be helpful.

Medications

Antibiotics are recommended if the infection/inflammation has exceeded 72 hours; the nipple is discharging pus or blood; signs and symptoms are sudden, severe, and bilateral or worsening fever and flulike symptoms persist; or the nipples are cracked, predisposing to bacteria entering the breast tissue.

8

Cardiovascular Health

CARDIOVASCULAR DISEASE

What Is It?

Cardiovascular disease is any disease of the heart and blood vessels. There are many types of cardiovascular diseases, including coronary artery disease (CAD), atherosclerosis, deep vein thrombosis, varicose veins, strokes, aneurysms, stenosis, and prolapse of the valves.

Who Gets It?

Men and women are both affected equally. Men are affected at approximately age 45, and women typically after age 55. It is the leading cause of death in women regardless of race.

Etiology

Coronary artery disease is the most common of all cardiovascular diseases and is caused by narrowing of the blood vessels from fat and cholesterol deposits (atherosclerosis). The result is diminished blood supply (including oxygen and nutrients) to the heart. Chest pain or angina occurs, and, in the event of a complete blockage of a portion of the coronary arteries, a heart attack occurs. (This frequently occurs as a result of a blood clot that forms within a previously narrowed artery.)

Cardiovascular disease is caused by a plethora of factors, including the following:

- Aging
- Hypertension
- Diabetes

- Smoking
- Lack of physical activity
- Being overweight or obese
- Family history of early heart disease (father or brother before age 55; mother or sister before age 65)
- Hypercholesterolemia (cholesterol less than 240 mg/dl and low-density lipoproteins [LDLs] less than 130 mg/dl) or low high-density lipoproteins (HDLs) (less than 40 mg/dl)

Technical Note

The human body needs cholesterol for a variety of functions, one of which is to help make the many hormones of the body. Cholesterol (a fat) is not soluble in the blood; to reach the various target organs, it is bound to a protein, forming a lipoprotein. Low-density lipoprotein (LDL) is called the "bad" cholesterol because it is the form in which cholesterol travels away from the liver to the various target organs, including the heart. High-density lipoprotein (HDL), the "good" cholesterol, is the form in which cholesterol is removed from target organs and blood vessels and transported back to the liver, where it is prepared for excretion. HDL helps keep cholesterol from building up in the walls of the arteries. The greater the levels of LDL in the bloodstream, the greater the risk of heart disease; the greater the levels of HDL in the blood, the lower the risk of heart disease.

Estrogen raises the HDL and lowers the LDL levels. Estrogen also helps prevent oxidation, making the LDLs less harmful to the blood vessels.

Signs and Symptoms

- Heart attack—nausea, sweating, light-headedness, vomiting, breathlessness; neck, shoulder, or abdominal discomfort; extreme fatigue or sleep disturbances
- Stroke—sudden loss of the use of an extremity, bladder or bowel incontinence, sudden weakness of the face, sudden visual disturbances, sudden dizziness, loss of balance or coordination, sudden severe headaches

Management

Lifestyle. The Mayo Clinic provides the following five preventive strategies for cardiovascular disease:

1. Risk factors should be assessed beginning at age 20, and every 5 years thereafter.
2. Smoking cessation. Tobacco smoke contains more than 4800 chemical substances, many of which can damage the heart and blood vessels, making them more prone to atherosclerosis. Nicotine in cigarette smoke makes the heart work harder by constricting blood vessels and increasing the heart rate and blood pressure. Carbon monoxide in cigarette smoke replaces some of the oxygen in the blood, which increases blood pressure by forcing the heart to work harder to supply enough oxygen. Smoking is the greatest risk factor for heart attack. Women who smoke are two to six times more likely to have a heart attack and are more likely to die after having a heart attack. Women who smoke and take birth control pills are 20 to 30 times more likely to have a heart attack or stroke when compared with women who do neither.
3. Exercise alone reduces the risk of cardiovascular disease by 30% to 50%. The heart is strengthened by the increased blood flow and subsequently can pump more blood with less effort; there is the added benefit of exercise to help control weight and manage conditions such as high blood pressure, diabetes, and hypercholesterolemia. Exercise also helps to reduce stress. Thirty to 60 minutes of moderately intense physical activity most days of the week is recommended.
4. Diet. Eating more grains, vegetables, and fruits, and limiting fat, especially saturated fat, can reduce the risk for heart disease. Saturated fat and trans fat increase the risk for CAD by raising blood cholesterol levels. Major sources of saturated fat include beef, butter, cheese, milk, and coconut and palm oil.
5. Five to seven servings of fruits and vegetables a day. Fruits and vegetables are highly effective in preventing cardiovascular disease. In addition, grains and legumes are full of cardiovascular disease–preventing nutrients. Soluble fiber, found in oatmeal, beans, apples, oranges, and grapefruit, may help lower blood cholesterol.

Supplementation

- Vitamin C and the carotenoids. Antioxidants help to prevent cholesterol from damaging the linings of the arteries, and the carotenoids keep cholesterol and fat deposits from being deposited in the blood vessels. These are found mainly in fruits and vegetables, such as green and red peppers, broccoli, brussels sprouts, leafy greens, tomatoes, strawberries, and oranges.

Clinical Pearl

The recommended daily allowance (RDA) for vitamin C is 75 mg in women and 90 mg in men. The American Journal of Clinical Nutrition *has stated that vitamin C is safe at dosages up to 2000 mg daily. Many authorities recommend higher dosages of vitamin C because of its utilization in multiple biosynthetic functions. In excess, vitamin C frequently will cause diarrhea.*

- Folate. The B vitamin known to prevent anemia of pregnancy and to aid fetal development has added benefits in helping to decrease homocysteine levels.
- Homocysteine is the amino acid normally found in the blood that when elevated is a risk factor for coronary heart disease and stroke. Elevated homocysteine levels also may impair endothelial vasomotor function, further affecting the ease by which blood flows through blood vessels. High levels of homocysteine may damage coronary arteries and make it easier for platelet aggregation to occur, predisposing to heart attack and stroke.
- A deficiency of folate, vitamin B_{12}, or vitamin B_6 may increase blood levels of homocysteine. Folate supplementation has been shown to decrease homocysteine levels and to improve endothelial function.
- Spinach, turnip greens and other green leafy vegetables, citrus fruits, dried beans, and peas are all natural sources of folate.
- Omega-3 fatty acids may decrease the risk of heart attack by providing protection against arrhythmia and lowering blood pressure levels. Omega-3 fatty acids can be found in fish, fish oils, flaxseed oil, and borage oil. Pregnant women should

avoid swordfish, king mackerel, tuna, and tile fish, which contain levels of mercury that might be harmful to the fetus.

- Manage obesity. Fatty tissue, like other tissue in the body, needs oxygen and nutrients. As weight increases, the amount of fat tissue increases, and the demand for oxygen and nutrients increases. This means the amount of blood circulating through the body also increases, which leads to added pressure on the arterial walls.

- Excess weight often is associated with an increased heart rate and a reduced capacity of the blood vessels to support blood. Excess weight also can lead to diabetes, high cholesterol, and high blood pressure, all of which increase the likelihood of heart disease.

Regular screening

- Regular blood pressure checks and lipid tests.

- Lipid profiles should be performed for the first time around age 20 and repeated every 5 years if it is within normal ranges. The lipid profile includes cholesterol and triglyceride (HDL and LDL) levels.

Clinical Pearl

- *Total cholesterol levels over 200 but less than 240 may not be of high risk if LDL levels are low and HDL levels are high. Women in the perimenopause frequently have slightly elevated total cholesterol levels and desirable HDL and LDL levels.*

- *HDL levels of 60 mg/dl or higher may protect against heart disease.*

- *HDL cholesterol levels of 40 mg/dl (1.04 mmol/L) or lower may increase the risk of developing heart disease, especially in the presence of high total cholesterol.*

- *Very high cholesterol and triglyceride levels may be caused by inherited forms of elevated cholesterol (hypercholesterolemia or hyperlipidemia).*

How to Calculate Body Mass Index without a Chart

1. Multiply the weight in pounds by 0.45.
2. Multiply height in inches by 0.025.
3. Square the answer from step 2.
4. Divide the answer from step 1 by the answer from step 3.

Patients with BMI over 27, and as low as 25, are at increased risk for health conditions such as cardiovascular disease, diabetes, and some cancers. See "Body Mass Index" table in Appendix.

9

Coccydynia

WHAT IS IT?

Coccydynia is pain in the coccyx.

WHO GETS IT?

Women and men of all ages. Coccydynia is more common in women.

ETIOLOGY

Coccydynia can be caused by direct trauma to the tailbone, typically from a fall resulting in irritation/inflammation to the ligaments of the sacrococcygeal articulation, disarticulation of the sacrococcygeal articulation, or fracture of the tailbone.

It can also be caused by childbirth, which can cause irritation, inflammation, or disarticulation of the sacrococcygeal articulation as the infant's head travels through the birth canal.

Signs and Symptoms

- Moderate to severe pain at the sacrum, coccyx, and surrounding tissues, sometimes accompanied by low back pain
- Pain worsens with prolonged sitting

Clinical Pearl

Because of the broader pelvis, women are more likely to sit on the coccyx as well as the ischial tuberosities, whereas men sit primarily on the ischial tuberosities. Women therefore experience more pain than men.

Diagnosis

- Presenting signs and symptoms
- History of fall or childbirth
- Digital rectal examination that reveals localized tenderness over the sacrococcygeal articulation and a misaligned coccyx
- Complete physical examination to rule out referred pain from the lumbosacral spine, lumbar disk herniation, tumors, and other pathology
- X-rays to rule out fracture or tumor
- Magnetic resonance imaging (MRI) in severe or nonimproving scenarios to rule out smaller tumors or localized infectious processes

Management

- Self-help
  - Donut pillow
  - Ice applied directly over the area of complaint

Spinal Manipulation

- Manipulation of the coccyx–internal and external coccygeal maneuvers are of benefit. In addition, use of the low force activator adjusting instrument has been demonstrated to provide relief.
- Manipulation of the sacrum and other pelvic structures may provide relief.

Physical Therapy

- Ultrasound over the sacrococcygeal articulation and ligaments

Massage Therapy

- Trigger point therapy to the levator ani and surrounding muscles may provide relief.
- Massaging or stretching the muscles attached to the coccyx has been shown to provide greater relief than manually moving the coccyx in some patients.

Medications

- Nonsteroidal anti-inflammatory drugs (NSAIDs)

Procedures

- Cortisone injections

10

Cultural Considerations

Cultural competence in women's health involves developing awareness, knowledge, and skills to optimize patient outcomes.

AWARENESS

Awareness is appreciation and acceptance of the myriad of interacting cultures that exist in any patient-provider encounter, including the following:

- The culture of the health care system (e.g., allopathy, alternative, natural, traditional Chinese medicine, chiropractic, naturopathy, homeopathy)
- Patients' inherent cultural beliefs about the health care system; about their own health; and about the cause, management, and outcomes of the condition or circumstance for which they are seeking treatment
- The provider's personal and professional cultural beliefs, including a code of ethics that affects his or her choices of health care delivery

KNOWLEDGE

An interest in and knowledge of some of these different cultural norms is predicated on the assumption that the patient-centered approach to health care warrants respectful consideration of the patient's belief systems even when they are in conflict with the provider's. The provider also acknowledges the potential for mutual learning that exists in the patient-provider encounter and purposefully learns differing worldviews.

Examples of differing views on health care include the following:

Cultural views on weight management

Obesity is evidence of affluence.	Obesity is a cause of illnesses.

Cultural views on disease

One disease—one cure.	One disease—multiple cures.
Only Allah has the cure for disease.	A medication may cure the disease.
There is a cure for every disease.	Many diseases are terminal.

Cultural views on exercise

Exercise is scheduled, deliberate, and purposeful.	Running aimlessly on a treadmill is incomprehensible; exercise happens as a result of daily activities.

Cultural views on preventive care

A visit to a health care provider is necessitated by illness.	A visit to a health care provider is necessary for screening procedures such as a Papanicolaou (Pap) smear.

Cultural views on health disclosure

Full disclosure is mandated by law.	Delivering bad news is taboo, and terminal outcomes are never discussed.

SKILLS

Failure to acknowledge differing worldviews potentially affects patient compliance and patient outcomes, hence the need for skill development. Skill development, as with all aspects of health care practice, is an ongoing process. Seeking out differing cultural encounters and recognizing the limitations inherent in some encounters are useful strategies. Interpreters, cultural brokers, community leaders, chaplains, and other healers are valuable resources.

Following are outlined select models for developing cultural competence.

Cultural Assessment

Perform a cultural assessment. Start with the LEARN model:

Try to assess where patients derive their ideas about disease and illness. Areas to consider include the following:

- Level of ethnic identity
- Use of informal network and supportive institutions in the ethnic/cultural community values orientation
- Language and communication process
- Migration experience
- Self-concept and self-esteem
- Influence of religion/spirituality on the belief system and behavior patterns
- Views and concerns about discrimination and institutional racism
- Views about the role that ethnicity plays
- Educational level and employment experiences
- Habits, customs, and beliefs
- Importance and impact associated with physical characteristics
- Cultural health beliefs and practices
- Current socioeconomic status

Ten Tips for Improving the Provider-Patient Relationship[*]

1. Do not necessarily treat the patient in the same manner you would want to be treated. Culture determines the roles for polite, caring behavior and will formulate the patient's concept of a satisfactory relationship.
2. Begin by being more formal with patients who were born in another culture. In most countries, a greater distance between caregiver and patient is maintained through the relationship. Except when treating children or very young adults, it is best to use the patient's last name when addressing him or her.

---

[*]From Salimbene S, Graczykowski JW: 10 tips for improving the caregiver/patient relationship across cultures. *When two cultures meet: American medicine and the cultures of diverse patient populations*, Book 1, *What language does your patient hurt in? An 8-part series of practical guides to the care and treatment of patients from other cultures*, Amherst, MA, 1995, Inter-Face International, Amherst Educational Publishing, pp 23–25.

3. Do not be insulted if the patient fails to look you in the eye or ask questions about treatment. In many cultures, it is disrespectful to look directly at another person (especially one in authority) or to make someone "lose face" by asking him or her questions.

4. Do not make any assumptions about the patient's ideas about the ways to maintain health, the cause of illness, or the means to prevent or cure it. Adopt a line of questioning that will help to determine some of the patient's central beliefs about health, illness, and illness prevention.

5. Allow the patient to be open and honest. Do not discount beliefs that are not held by Western biomedicine. Often, patients are afraid to tell Western caregivers that they are visiting a folk healer or are taking an alternative medicine concurrently with Western treatment because in the past they have experienced ridicule.

6. Do not discount the possible effects of beliefs in the supernatural on the patient's health. If the patient believes that the illness has been caused by embrujado (bewitchment), the evil eye, or punishment, the patient is not likely to take any responsibility for his or her cure. Belief in the supernatural may result in his or her failure to either follow medical advice or comply with the treatment plan.

7. Inquire indirectly about the patient's belief in the supernatural or use of nontraditional cures. Say something like, "Many of my patients from __ believe, do, or visit __. Do you?"

8. Try to ascertain the value of involving the entire family in the treatment. In many cultures, medical decisions are made by the immediate family or the extended family. If the family can be involved in the decision-making process and the treatment plan, there is a greater likelihood of gaining the patient's compliance with the course of treatment.

9. Be restrained in relating bad news or explaining in detail complications that may result from a particular course of treatment. "The need to know" is a unique American trait. In many cultures, placing oneself in the doctor's hands represents an act of trust and a desire to transfer the responsibility for treatment to the physician. Watch for and respect signs that the patient has learned as much as he or she is able to deal with.

10. Whenever possible, incorporate into the treatment plan the
    patient's folk medication and folk beliefs that are not specif-
    ically contraindicated. This will encourage the patient to
    develop trust in the treatment and will help to ensure that
    the treatment plan is followed.

11

Diabetes and Insulin Resistance

INSULIN RESISTANCE

Insulin resistance is caused by failure of the cells to respond adequately to stimulus from insulin; this initiates a vicious cycle in which blood sugar levels rise and, in response, the pancreas accelerates insulin production. The cells eventually respond and glucose in the blood enters the cells en masse, resulting in a corresponding rapid drop in blood sugar levels and a hypoglycemic state. As simple carbohydrates and foods with a high glycemic index are ingested, the cycle repeats until, eventually, the pancreas is overextended and no longer able to produce sufficient amounts of insulin, and diabetes results. Insulin resistance is marked by simultaneous elevations of blood sugars and blood insulin.

- The liver responds to the elevated blood sugar levels by rapidly converting the excess sugars to fat.
- Glucose from sugars is converted to energy in the cells; in the absence of this critical source of energy, fatigue and food cravings result.
- The excess fat cells result in increased hormone load as more estrogen is stored in fatty tissue and synthesized via the aromatase enzyme.
- Aromatase enzyme synthesizes estrogen via the androstenedione pathway, which ultimately may result in excess testosterone.
- Insulin resistance is a prediabetic condition.

SYNDROME X

Syndrome X, also called *metabolic syndrome,* is a cluster of symptoms that predispose to heart disease. It is defined by the National Cholesterol Education Program as the presence of any three of the following:

- Excess weight around the waist (waist measurement of more than 40 inches for men and more than 35 inches for women)
- High levels of triglycerides (150 mg/dl or higher)
- Low levels of high-density lipoprotein (HDL) cholesterol (below 40 mg/dl for men and below 50 mg/dl for women)
- High blood pressure (130/85 mm Hg or higher)
- High fasting blood glucose levels (110 mg/dl or higher)

DIABETES

Adult-onset diabetes, also known as type 2 diabetes, is caused by inadequate response of the body to insulin and inadequate production of insulin by the pancreas.

Etiology

- Stress
- Diet
- Being overweight
- Family history of diabetes
- Low HDL and high triglycerides
- High blood pressure
- History of gestational diabetes
- Genetics/hereditary factors
- History of giving birth to babies weighing more than 9 pounds
- A person from one of the following groups:
  - African American
  - American Indian
  - Hispanic/Latino
  - Asian American/Pacific Islander

Signs and Symptoms

- Excessive thirst
- Fatigue following high-carbohydrate meals

- Increased abdominal weight gain
- Extreme fatigue after eating foods with a high glycemic index

Diagnostic Protocols

Blood tests

- Fasting glucose levels of 126 mg/dl or higher on more than one test are evidence of diabetes. Levels of 100 to 125 mg/dl indicate impaired fasting glucose and suggest a prediabetic or insulin resistance state.
- The glucose tolerance test (the patient is required to fast overnight and be evaluated 2 hours after drinking a sweet liquid). Insulin resistance or a prediabetic state is suspected if the blood glucose is between 140 and 199 mg/dl 2 hours after drinking the sweet liquid, and diabetes is indicated if the levels are over 200 mg/dl.
- Hemoglobin A_{1c} assay readings over 7% indicate diabetes or poor diabetic control.
- The euglycemic clamp, which is a complicated and expensive test.

Management

Lifestyle. A diet based on the American Diabetes Association (ADA) recommendations and a low-fat vegan diet have been demonstrated to improve glycemic and lipid control in type 2 diabetics. Whole grains and foods high in magnesium are important components of the diet. Select recommendations include all legumes, most vegetables, brown rice instead of white rice, whole fruits instead of fruit juices, blackstrap molasses or sugar substitutes instead of white sugar, foods with a low glycemic index, garlic, onions, olives, mangoes, and nuts.

Exercise. Researchers at the National Institutes of Health diabetes prevention program found that lifestyle changes reduced the risk of diabetes by 58%, far better than the 31% improvement noted with prediabetic drugs such as metformin. They concluded that the most effective way to reduce the risk of diabetes is to be active and have a low-calorie, low-fat diet.

Body mass index. Maintaining a body mass index (BMI) of less than 24 (see Appendix) and a waist-to-hip ratio of 1.0 or less in men and 0.8 or less in women can reduce the risk of developing diabetes.

Clinical Pearl

Patients who are very athletic may have a high BMI, but have low body fat. These individuals may benefit from a body fat analysis. A low BMI does not necessarily mean low body fat. BMI and waist-to-hip ratio should be used concurrently.

Nutritional recommendations/supplementation

- Cinnamon 1 g/day in split doses (approximately 1/2 teaspoon) has been shown to reduce blood sugar levels in diabetics. In studies, the 1 g dosage appeared to be the ideal dosage to maintain lowered blood sugar levels after intake was removed. The higher dosages did not maintain the same lowered blood sugar levels.
- Use xylitol instead of sugar as a sweetening alternative. Xylitol has a low glycemic index, has minimal effect on blood sugar and insulin levels, and reduces carbohydrate cravings and binge eating.
- Chromium 500 to 1000 mcg daily increases the ability of the cells to burn fat instead of glucose.
- Eicosapentaenoic acid and docosahexaenoic acid (EPA/DHA).
- B-complex vitamins.

Medications

- Biguanides such as metformin (Glucophage) improve insulin responsiveness.
- Thiazolidinediones such as troglitazone (which has been withdrawn from the market because of increased risk of liver toxicity) improve insulin responsiveness and have been shown to delay or prevent type 2 diabetes in Hispanic women with a history of gestational diabetes.
- Alpha-glucosidase inhibitors such as acarbose restrict or delay the absorption of carbohydrates after eating, resulting in a slower rise of blood glucose levels.
- Sulfonylureas and meglitinides increase insulin production.
- Intensive insulin management includes continuous subcutaneous insulin infusion or daily injections.

Additional Screening/Monitoring Procedures

- Blood pressure
- Lipid management

- Ocular examination
- Screening for renal disease
- Peripheral vascular examination and a foot examination (including evaluation for and management of foot ulcers and infections)

How to Calculate Body Mass Index without a Chart

1. Multiply the weight in pounds by 0.45.
2. Multiply height in inches by 0.025.
3. Square the answer from step 2.
4. Divide the answer from step 1 by the answer from step 3.
   Refer also to the "Body Mass Index" table in the Appendix.

12

Domestic Violence

WHAT IS IT?

Domestic violence is also known as intimate partner violence (IPV), abuse, and violence experienced in intimate relationships. The abuse can be physical, mental, or emotional.

WHO IS ABUSED?

- IPV occurs across all socioeconomic, gender, racial, ethnic, age, ideological, cultural, and spiritual barriers.
- IPV occurs in both opposite-sex and same-sex relationships.
- IPV happens to both men and women; however, more women are abused than men. Data from the Bureau of Justice suggest that women in their late teens to early twenties are more likely than older women to be victims of domestic violence from a husband, boyfriend, or former partner, and that older women, i.e., ages 35 to 45, were more likely to be murdered by their intimate partners, because they were vulnerable for longer periods of time.
- IPV can escalate during pregnancy.
- Abuse and violence experienced by women in intimate relationships is a health concern that affects approximately one in nine American women and as many as one in four pregnant women.

ETIOLOGY

The myriad of causes for IPV include issues with control and a historical failure in society to acknowledge IPV as a health care concern and not solely as a private matter.

SIGNS AND SYMPTOMS/PRESENTING COMPLAINTS

- Migraines
- Chronic headaches
- Bruises
- Neck pain
- Back pain
- Anxiety disorders
- Muscle tension
- Digestive complaints
- Dysfunctional menstrual bleeding caused by stress
- Depression
- Eating disorders
- Chest pain
- Tingling and numbness
- Pelvic pain
- Arrhythmia
- Urinary tract infections and vaginitis
- Ear pain or evidence of a ruptured tympanic membrane
- Dyspareunia or evidence of rectal or genital injury
- Bruises on the face, neck, or abdomen
- Bruises on the arm
- Centrally located injuries involving the buttocks, breasts, body, and genital region (the "bathing suit pattern")
- Injuries involving the head and neck
- Defensive posture injuries, which may involve the palms, the small finger side of the forearm, the back, and the back of the head

DIAGNOSIS

- By signs and symptoms
- History and physical examination

INTIMATE PARTNER VIOLENCE SCREENING

Health care providers are uniquely positioned to screen for domestic violence in a private setting and point their patients to resources that empower them to work their way out of the domestic violence cycle.

It is recommended that health care providers screen all adult female patients for IPV, and incorporate IPV screening into the general intake. Furthermore, it is important that health care providers screen for IPV whenever

- Patients report to the emergency department for complaints associated with trauma
- The cause given for the injury does not support the type of injury
- Fractures and injuries in various stages of healing are observed
- A delay has occurred in the patient's seeking medical attention
- The patient demonstrates visible signs of depression

Technical Note

IPV should be suspected whenever the

- Partner appears controlling
- Partner attempts to answer all questions for the patient
- Partner insists on being present while care is being offered to the patient
- Patient fails to make eye contact

It is equally important to note that some of these types of behaviors are cultural norms and are not necessarily indicative of IPV. The health care provider should attempt to ask the patient when her partner is not close by if she would like her partner to be present during the office visit. IPV screening should never occur in the presence of the partner.

Sample screening questions include the following:

- "How are things at home?"
- "Do you feel safe at home?"
- "Has your partner ever physically hurt you?"
- "Are you afraid of your partner?"
- "Do you feel your partner tries to control you?"
- "Has your partner ever forced you into a sexual act that you did not wish to participate in?"
- "Are you in danger?"
- "Does your partner hit you when he (or she) is angry?"

Screening questions may be preceded by an introductory comment such as the following:

- "There are certain questions that I ask all my patients because we know, from statistical data, that many women are or have been victims of domestic violence."
- "Some of my patients are in relationships where they are afraid their partners may hurt them."

Once domestic violence has been identified, it is important that the provider validate the victim as the victim and not the perpetrator. It is equally important that the provider does not minimize the victim's experience. Sample responses include the following:

- "I believe you."
- "You are not alone."
- "This situation must be very difficult for you."
- "The violence is not your fault and only (name of abuser) can choose to stop this behavior."
- "Your safety concerns me," or, "I am concerned for your safety."
- "No one deserves to be abused."
- "You have options."
- "There are resources available."

The health care provider should point the patient to available resources, assist as needed in following up with the resources (domestic violence shelters, advocacy groups, etc.), and encourage and facilitate the preparation of an exit plan. The exit plan involves identifying resources (friends, family, neighbors, etc.) who can be called on to assist in the event of an imminent exit from the home, and locating a safe place to store critical items such as the children's favorite toys, any essential medications, and cash.

MANAGEMENT

Once domestic violence has been identified, the health care provider should

- Validate the individual's story.
- Remind the individual that she or he is not at fault and that no one deserves to be abused.
- Ascertain whether there are children involved and whether they are at risk.
- Follow all state guidelines for reporting if there are children at risk (health care providers are mandated to report if they are made aware of violence to children).

- Provide resources—domestic violence shelters, reading materials, local advocacy agencies, and even the police.
- Follow state guidelines for reporting abuse when the victim is an adult. Most states do not mandate reporting if the abuse is perpetrated against an adult (many states make an exception if there are weapons involved or the adult is classified as a "vulnerable adult"), and several advocacy groups do not recommend the provider's reporting on behalf of the victim.
- Document all examination findings in as much detail as possible.

Clinical Pearl

What can be done to prevent domestic violence?
- *If abuse is suspected—ask.*
- *If abuse is confirmed, voice concern, listen to the individual's story, and validate her or his experience.*
- *Discretion is critical. The abuse should not be discussed with others without permission.*
- *Empower the patient by commenting on the courage and strength that it takes to survive domestic violence.*
- *Provide resources.*
- *Be mindful of personal safety.*
- *Be clear about the role of the health care provider, and avoid becoming inappropriately involved.*

WHY DO WOMEN STAY IN ABUSIVE RELATIONSHIPS?

The reasons why women stay are multiple and varied and include the following:
- Finances
- Fear of the abuser
- Concern about the welfare of the children
- Commitment to the abuser
- Love for the abuser
- Lack of self-esteem
- Fear that the abuser might hurt himself or herself

- Fear that the abuser might hurt the children or the victim herself or himself
- Fear for the welfare of a beloved pet

WHY DO ABUSERS ABUSE?

The reasons are multiple and varied and include the following:
- Learned behavior—many abusers were themselves abused as children
- Lack of self-esteem
- Poor coping skills
- Substance abuse
- The need to control

13

Dysmenorrhea

WHAT IS IT?

- Dysmenorrhea—painful menses:
  - Primary dysmenorrhea is painful menses that is not related to any definable pelvic lesion. Primary dysmenorrhea begins with the first ovulatory cycles in women under age 20, and in most women resolves or subsides by age 30, with the onset of sexual activity, or with childbirth.
  - Secondary dysmenorrhea is painful menses that is related to the presence of pelvic lesions or pelvic disease (e.g., endometriosis, fibroids, episiotomy, and pelvic inflammatory disease).

WHO GETS IT?

Most female adolescents and young adults get dysmenorrhea. It is the most common reason for absences from school and work.

ETIOLOGY

Primary

- Increased uterine activity/forceful contractions
  - The uterus contracts to expel menstrual blood; the force of the contractions can temporarily cause ischemia by occluding uterine blood supply.
  - Excessive production of vasopressin causes contraction of the smooth muscle of the uterus and the small muscles within the blood vessels. Excess vasopressin can stimulate very powerful contractions, which increases pain.

    Vasopressin is formed in the supraoptic and paraventricular nuclei of the hypothalamus and is transported to the posterior lobe through the hypothalamohypophysial tract.

- Overproduction of prostaglandins. Prostaglandins are a group of chemicals, some of which are formed locally at the endometrium. Like vasopressin, some prostaglandins cause smooth muscle contractions. Overproduction of prostaglandins can cause platelet aggregation, vasoconstriction, intense and irregular contractions, and ischemia.

Technical Note

Prostaglandins are not stored in the tissues, they are produced locally (in situ) from arachidonic acid and other fatty acids during the luteal phase of the menstrual cycle. Inflammatory prostaglandins include prostaglandin E_2 (PGE_2); antiinflammatory prostaglandins include PGE_1 and PGE_3.

- Cervical stenosis. The cervical os is narrow in nonparous females. The expulsion of a nonliquefied clot through a narrowed cervical os is a potential cause of pain. Parous females can experience pain from the expulsion of a large nonliquefied clot. Women have described clots the size of a plum and larger.
- The uterus is situated in the middle of the pelvis, between the symphysis pubis and the sacrum. Misalignment of the pelvic girdle, including the sacrum and ilia, can cause dysmenorrhea.
- The uterus is supported within the pelvic cavity by the two broad ligaments, the two round ligaments, and the two uterosacral ligaments, as well as other ligaments. Imbalance of the tension within the ligaments can predispose to dysmenorrhea.
- The uterus receives its innervation from spinal nerves T12–L4 and S2–S4. Misalignment in the vertebrae that encase the exiting spinal nerves at these levels causes interference, which can affect the function of the uterus and result in dysmenorrhea.
- Psychosocial and constitutional factors such as diabetes, anemia, stress, and learned behavior are all possible causes for dysmenorrhea, either because of a lower pain threshold or increased sensitivity to pain.

Secondary

- Postsurgical adhesions caused by caesarian section, episiotomy, or tearing with birth.

- Cervical stenosis occurring after surgical procedures to the cervix.
- Trigger points in the muscles that alter tension and the normal dynamics of the uterus.
- The intrauterine device (IUD) is a contraceptive device that works by irritating the endometrium, thereby hindering implantation. This local irritation may predispose to dysmenorrhea.
- Endometriosis, a condition characterized by the presence of endometrial tissue outside the uterus, causes local inflammation, scar tissue, and pain.
- Fibroids are benign tumors of the uterus that cause pain by creating inflammation in the uterus and placing direct pressure on the spine.
- Pelvic inflammatory disease (PID) frequently results in scar tissue in the endometrial and abdominal cavities and subsequent predisposition to dysmenorrhea.

SIGNS AND SYMPTOMS

Primary

Dull, midline, cramping, or spasmodic lower abdominal pain begins shortly before or at the onset of menses and may radiate to the lower back or the inner thighs. Ancillary symptoms include nausea, diarrhea, vomiting, headache, anxiety, and fatigue.

Secondary

A dull ache in the lower abdomen may begin several hours to several days before the onset of menses, and frequently is accompanied by headache, lower back pain, depression, and fatigue. The duration of secondary amenorrhea depends on the cause. In some cases it may begin with ovulation and extend for 2 weeks through the next menses.

MANAGEMENT

Lifestyle

- Rest. Tense muscles contract more forcefully. Relaxed muscles contract with less intensity.
- Exercise tones the muscles of the pelvic floor and the core abdominal muscles and releases pressure on the articular

facets in the lumbar spine. These include knee/chest stretches and core abdominal strengthening.

- Correction of poor posture. A swayback is a cause of strain to the pelvic muscles, which aggravates dysmenorrhea.
- Kegel exercises involve deep pelvic floor contractions to tone the levator ani muscles (see Appendix). The levator ani is composed of the pubococcygeus, puborectalis, and iliococcygeus muscles.
- Heat packs on the abdomen will relax the muscles of the uterus.
- Orgasm. This draws blood to the muscles of the pelvis, and this aids with relaxation and decreases pain.
- Childbirth increases uterine vascularity, which enables the uterine muscles to relax.
- Direct pressure over the neurolymphatic points with corollaries to the uterus and ovaries. These are bilateral points situated anteriorly on the pubic bone just lateral to the symphysis pubis and posteriorly on the lamina of the second, third, and fourth lumbar vertebrae.

Nutritional Supplementation

- Calcium 1200 to 1800 mg/day; dietary sources include dairy, green leafy vegetables, broccoli, and sardines
- Magnesium 500 mg/day; dietary sources include green leafy vegetables, molasses, soybeans, dairy, and some nuts and seeds
- EPA/DHA Eicosapentaenoic acid and docosahexaenoic acid (EPA/DHA) 400 to 1000 mg/day
- Red raspberry leaf tea, which aids in improving or maintaining healthy functioning of the reproductive organs

Technical Note

Raspberry leaf tea may inhibit the absorption of iron.

Diet

The following foods should be ingested sparingly:
- Red meats and dairy—precursors to the inflammatory prostaglandins via arachidonic acid

- Alcohol—a liver stressor that may impair functioning of the detoxification pathways
- Caffeine—a sympathetic nervous system stimulant that can intensify smooth muscle contractions of the uterus

---

Technical Note

The levator ani is supplied by a branch from the fourth sacral nerve and by a branch that is derived from the perineal or sometimes from the inferior hemorrhoidal division of the pudendal nerve. The coccygeus is supplied by a branch from the fourth and fifth sacral nerves. The muscles within the pelvis include the obturator internus and the piriformis, which are muscles of the lower extremity, and the levator ani and coccygeus, which together form the pelvic diaphragm and are associated with the pelvic viscera.

SPINAL AND PELVIC MANIPULATION

- Any misalignment of the pelvis should be corrected. In particular, the sacrum, symphysis pubis, and coccyx, which are primary attachment points for the levator ani and coccygeus muscles, should be assessed for misalignments.

Clinical Pearl

Sacrum subluxations are prominent findings in dysmenorrhea, including rotation, and a base anterior or nutated sacrum.

Technical Note

If the patient is unable to perform a squat beyond 90 degrees when the feet are shoulder width apart or has to raise the heels off the ground in order to perform the squat, there is probable cause for a sacrum restriction in nutation.

- Leg length discrepancies should be addressed to aid stabilization of the pelvis and reduce any strain on the piriformis and obturator muscles.

PHYSICAL THERAPY

Transcutaneous electrical nerve stimulation (TENS) is a modality that uses electrical impulses to interrupt pain signals.

MUSCLE THERAPY

The muscles of the pelvic girdle and abdomen are assessed for trigger points and hypertonicity.

LYMPHATIC DRAINAGE

The sacral pump and other lymphatic drainage techniques may be used.

Technical Note

In the sacral pump technique, the sacrum is tractioned caudally and pumped two or three times. This can be repeated for up to five cycles.

Neurolymphatic treatment points for dysmenorrhea are as follows:

- Anterior: upper edges of the pubic bone just lateral to the symphysis pubis
- Posterior: L2–L4 lamina
- Organ correlation: uterus and ovaries

MEDICATIONS

Primary Dysmenorrhea

- Nonsteroidal antiinflammatory drugs (NSAIDs)
- Oral contraceptives

Secondary Dysmenorrhea

- Pain management
- Management of the underlying cause

14

Dyspareunia

WHAT IS IT?

Dyspareunia is painful sexual intercourse.

WHO GETS IT?

Sexually active women of all ages can get dyspareunia.

ETIOLOGY

Biomechanical Factors

The pelvic floor is composed of nine muscles in three layers, which form a sling hinged on the anterior surface by the pubic bones and on the posterior surface by the coccyx. Within this sling of muscles is the opening for the vagina, the anus/rectum, and the urethra. Any change to the biomechanics of the pelvic girdle can result in dyspareunia. In addition, the sacral plexus lies on the piriformis and may be affected by injuries or biomechanical factors that cause piriformis strain.

- The levator ani consists of the pubococcygeus, puborectalis, and iliococcygeus muscles. It is supplied by the fourth sacral nerve and by a branch derived from the perineal or sometimes from the inferior hemorrhoidal division of the pudendal nerve. The coccygeus is supplied by the fourth and fifth sacral nerves. Irritation to these nerves from pathologic and biomechanical forces may predispose to dyspareunia.
- Postural alterations. The support of the pelvis is controlled by the larger gluteus maximus, medius, piriformis, psoas, and transversus abdominal muscles. When these are weakened by factors such as poor posture, some of the smaller muscles,

including the levator ani, are recruited to help stabilize the pelvis. This is not their primary function and, as a result, they rapidly become strained, leading to pain, inflammation, trigger point formation, and vaginismus.

- Spinal misalignments. Alterations of the biomechanical integrity of the spine can cause irritation of the nerves that supply the pelvis, reproductive tract organs, and vagina. This can ultimately cause dyspareunia.

Pregnancy and Delivery

- Pregnancy and childbirth may cause alterations in the tone of the core abdominal muscles. Maintaining posture necessitates recruiting the smaller muscles of the pelvis, which are not equipped for this task. The result is muscle inflammation, strain, and the development of trigger points. Several of these muscles support the vagina.
  - Episiotomy/tearing of the perineum during vaginal birth also can cause scar tissue, which results in soft tissue hypomobility.
  - Nerve supply to the pelvic girdle may be impaired by damage during delivery, causing dyspareunia.
  - Postpartum changes. As many as 40% of women report problems with sexual activity 3 months after birth, and 20% 12 months after birth. Almost half of all breast-feeding women report some problems with sexual activity. The elevated prolactin and decreased estrogen state that occurs with breast-feeding predisposes to vaginal dryness, fragility in the epithelial tissue of the vaginal vault, and ultimately dyspareunia.

Tipped or Retroverted Uterus

A tipped or retroverted uterus alters the position of the cervix in the vaginal vault, and this may cause dyspareunia.

Drug Side Effects

Medications such as those used for allergies, hypertension, and depression may affect amounts of vaginal lubrication, causing vaginal dryness and dyspareunia.

Psychosocial/Psychologic Factors

Issues such as depression; substance abuse; expectations, attitudes, and fears about sexuality; partner expectations; previous or current domestic or sexual abuse; and gender role expectations all may cause vaginismus, which in turn causes dyspareunia.

Stress and Anxiety

Muscles respond to stress and anxiety by becoming tense, hypertonic, and contracted. Contracted muscles do not stretch, causing pain. Vaginismus is painful spasming of the vagina as a result of contraction of the muscles surrounding the vagina.

Inflammation and Infection

The deep fascia of the perineum is connected to the fascia surrounding the levator ani muscles, coccygeus muscles, and pelvic viscera. Inflammation or infection of any of these intertwined structures in the pelvic girdle can cause dyspareunia. Conditions that cause inflammation or infection include the following:
- Ovarian cysts
- Pelvic inflammatory disease (PID)
- Endometriosis
- Fibroids
- Fibromyalgia
- Irritable bowel syndrome (IBS)

Pelvic Adhesions and Trigger Points

Pelvic adhesions and trigger points can cause local and referred pain.

Vulvodynia

See Chapter 34.

Menopause

With menopause comes a decline in estrogen and other hormones. A function of estrogen is to maintain the integrity of epithelial tissues and to facilitate lubrication of the vaginal vault. In menopause, the vagina may not receive adequate lubrication, and the tissues atrophy, resulting in petechial hemorrhaging of the vaginal vault and a condition known as atrophic vaginitis (see section on atrophic vaginitis).

Trauma

Past or present injury such as trauma to the tailbone or groin from a fall, sports activity such as horseback riding, or gymnastics can result in dyspareunia.

Coccydynia

See Chapter 9.

Constipation

Constipation can lead to dyspareunia when impacted stools create pressure on the rectum and vagina.

SIGNS AND SYMPTOMS

- Painful intercourse
- Pelvic or vaginal heaviness
- Backache
- Rectal pain with vaginal penetration
- Involuntary vaginal spasms

Clinical Pearl

- *Pain with initial penetration may suggest vaginismus, trigger points in the pelvic diaphragm, or scars of episiotomy.*
- *Pain with deep penetration may suggest infections, endometriosis, ovarian cysts, fibroids, trigger points in the abdominal muscles, or pudendal nerve dysfunction.*
- *Pain with either initial or deep penetration or both may suggest pudendal nerve dysfunction, pelvic misalignments, infection, scars of episiotomy, trauma, and any irritation of the fascia.*

DIAGNOSIS

Diagnosis is based on symptoms and on screening tests for any of the conditions described previously.

MANAGEMENT

Lifestyle and Self-Help Strategies

- Help should be sought. Far too many women live for years with the pain of dyspareunia instead of consulting with a women's health care provider.
- Postpartum. Exercises to strengthen the core and pelvic outlet (e.g., pelvic tilt) may relieve dyspareunia.
- Kegel exercises draw blood to the region, increase tone of flaccid muscles, and relax spasmed muscles.
- Self-massage or partner massage of the perineum with vitamin E oil, flaxseed oil, or castor oil may relieve dyspareunia.
- Gentle stretches of the vaginal orifice by inserting the thumb into the vaginal opening and stretching the lower border from superior to inferior may relieve dyspareunia. (Stretching can be performed by oneself or by a partner.) The thumb is inserted into the vaginal vault and downward pressure is applied at the 5-, 6-, and 7-o'clock positions until a slight burning sensation is felt. Two to three repetitions are performed daily.
- Dilators come in graduated sizes and are used in place of the fingers to stretch the vaginal vault and treat trigger points.
- Hot and cold packs to the lower abdomen and pelvic diaphragm.
- Postural mindfulness.
- Exercises to strengthen the core.
- Counseling for psychosocial and psychosexual concerns.

SPINAL AND PELVIC MANIPULATION

Women with dyspareunia should be assessed and treated for spinal and pelvic misalignments.

MUSCLE THERAPY

- Trigger point therapy to any affected muscle groups
- Myofascial and scar tissue release techniques

- Massage of the perineum, abdominal cavity, and gluteal muscles
- Systemic massage for relaxation
- Visceral mobilization

PHYSICAL THERAPY

- Biofeedback
- Electrical therapies to the pelvic floor
- Internal and external myofascial release
- Postpartum massage of the perineum beginning 2 to 3 weeks postpartum to minimize the risk of adhesions

MEDICATIONS

- Estrogen creams for dyspareunia caused by atrophic vaginitis

---

Clinical Pearl

Prolonged, frequent use of Vitamin E or castor oil is not recommended because there is some risk of clogging the pores.

15

Endometriosis

WHAT IS IT?

Endometriosis is the growth of endometrial tissue in ectopic sites (Figure 15-1). The endometrium is the inner lining of the uterus. In endometriosis, uterine cells migrate or develop abnormally in ectopic sites such as the ovaries, bladder, cervix, rectum, neck, upper arm, and axillary area. This endometrial tissue responds to hormones as if in the uterus, proliferating and multiplying during the first half of the cycle, and imbibing, specializing, and disintegrating after ovulation. The result is bleeding, inflammation, scar formation, adhesions, deformity, infertility, and pain, which is often debilitating.

WHO GETS IT?

Endometriosis occurs in menstruating females during their reproductive years and frequently is diagnosed in the midtwenties to early thirties.

ETIOLOGY

The etiology of endometriosis is not fully understood. Proposed causes include the following:

Retrograde Menstruation

The theory of retrograde menstruation is that a narrow uterine outlet can cause blood to pool in the uterus, resulting in backflow out of the fallopian tubes into the abdominal cavity.

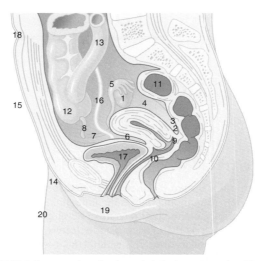

FIGURE 15-1 Common sites of endometriosis in decreasing order of frequency: (1) ovary, (2) cul-de-sac, (3) uterosacral ligaments, (4) broad ligaments, (5) fallopian tubes, (6) uterovesical fold, (7) round ligaments, (8) vermiforma appendix, (9) vagina, (10) rectovaginal septum, (11) rectosigmoid colon, (12) cecum, (13) ileum, (14) inguinal canals, (15) abdominal scars, (16) ureters, (17) urinary bladder, (18) umbilicus, (19) vulva, and (20) peripheral sites. (From Hacker NF, Moore JG, Gambone JC: *Essentials of obstetrics and gynecology,* ed 4, Philadelphia, 2004, WB Saunders.)

Some have suggested that the use of tampons and antifungal creams may contribute to endometriosis by delaying the expulsion of menstrual blood, thereby causing pooling and backflow.

Hereditary Factors

There is growing evidence of a familial or genetic cause for endometriosis. The European Society for Human Reproduction and Embryology published a study providing further evidence that there is a genetic link to endometriosis. In the study conducted on 750 women in Iceland who had a surgical diagnosis of endometriosis between 1981 and 1993, they found that a woman has more than five times the normal risk of developing endometriosis if her sister has the disease, and that even having a cousin with endometriosis raises a woman's risk by more than 50%.

Lymphatic and Vascular Flow (Halban's Theory)

Endometrial tissue has been identified in distal sites, including the neck, arms, and feet. This suggests that endometrial tissue may travel via blood and lymph channels.

Coelomic Epithelium

Mucous membranes of the uterus, fallopian tubes, ovaries, vagina, external ovarian lining, and internal lining of the pelvis are all derived embryologically from coelomic epithelium. This theory suggests that coelomic epithelium may differentiate abnormally in these sites.

SIGNS AND SYMPTOMS

- Pain in any or all of the pelvic organs
- Dysmenorrhea
- Dyspareunia
- Mittelschmerz (pain at ovulation)
- Spotting/bleeding—intermenstrual spotting or bleeding
- Infertility
- Low back pain

Clinical Pearl

The severity of the disease does not necessarily correlate with the severity of symptoms.

DIAGNOSIS

Diagnosis requires a detailed history, which might elicit any one or several of the following:
- History of infertility
- Moderate to severe menstrual cramps
- Pain with intercourse
- Abnormal bleeding patterns
- Constipation
- Pain with bowel movements
- Bloating and abdominal swelling

A pelvic examination also is performed:

- The pelvic examination may be painful and reveal a uterus that is retroverted, rigid, or not freely moveable; palpable nodules in the uterosacral ligaments; and cystic ovarian enlargements.
- The speculum examination may reveal the presence of endometriomas, which are blue, domelike bulges in the vagina and cervix.
- Definitive diagnosis of endometriosis requires either laparoscopy or magnetic resonance imaging (MRI). In the laparoscopic evaluation, carbon dioxide gas is infused into the abdomen, causing distention. This enables the structures to be visualized better. A scope is inserted into the abdomen through an incision made in the navel, and the presence of scar tissue, adhesions, chocolate ovarian cysts, and powder burn lesions provides evidence of endometriosis. In addition, the patency of the fallopian tubes can be determined.

MANAGEMENT

- Self-help

Diet

- Decrease refined sugars and simple carbohydrates. Insulin resistance results in elevated levels of estrogen, which worsens the symptoms of endometriosis. Insulin resistance can occur under conditions of prolonged stress and with high-carbohydrate diets.
- Eliminate caffeine.
- Increase dietary fiber. Whole grains in the form of oats, rice, buckwheat, and millet are excellent sources. They enhance the function of the elimination pathways and provide B vitamins, which are useful in the body's synthesis of the anti-inflammatory prostaglandins.
- Avoid meats, dairy, and poultry from hormone-fattened livestock. These are exogenous sources of estrogens. Red meats and dairy increase systemic production of arachidonic acid, a precursor to the inflammatory prostaglandins.
- Increase intake of all phytoestrogens, particularly the cruciferous vegetables kale, collard greens, cauliflower, cabbage, broccoli, and brussels sprouts, which are sources of calcium and indole-3 carbinol, a necessary precursor in the synthesis of the

"weaker" 2-OH estrogens. Increase intake of legumes, including lentils, chickpeas, and mung beans, and soy products, such as tofu, tempeh, and other soybeans.

- Fruits such as kiwi, figs, raspberries, and oranges are useful adjuncts in the management of endometriosis as they are sources of calcium, magnesium, and potassium, which help to relax the muscles and decrease menstrual pain and cramping.

Psychosocial Factors

Stress causes a rise in cortisol, which affects other hormones such as estrogen. Attending to psychosocial factors is essential to the management of endometriosis.

Acupressure

Apply gentle, direct pressure over acupressure points for general reproductive health as follows: spleen 6, located about three to four finger widths above the medial malleolus; hoku hand point at the junction of the thumb and index finger.

Acupuncture

Acupuncture may relieve pain and pelvic congestion. Ren (zhen) 4 is midway between the navel and pubic bone, and du 4 is directly over L2. In traditional Chinese medicine (TCM), these points would be treated concurrently with moxibustion, a warm heat source from burning herbs or needling.

Spinal Manipulation

Specific spinal adjustments to the thoracolumbar spine and sacrum may alleviate biomechanical distortions and decrease nerve interference.

Massage/Myofascial Release

Low back and abdominal massage may be helpful. Abdominal massage techniques that break up scar tissue, release trigger points, and "free" the uterus are particularly beneficial.

Heat pack application over the abdomen is useful, either by itself or along with castor oil or vitamin E oil application as a precursor to myofascial release techniques.

Physical Therapy

- Exercises with special emphasis on increasing core strength deficits are beneficial
- Comprehensive musculoskeletal examination and treatment to address muscular imbalances in the pelvis, hips, and pelvic floor
- Electrical therapies, including transcutaneous electrical nerve stimulation (TENS)

Medications

- Birth control pills. The hormones in either the minipill or the combined pill diminish the intensity of endometrial symptoms by inhibiting growth of endometrial tissue.
- Nonsteroidal anti-inflammatory drugs (NSAIDs) such as Motrin, Anaprox, and Naprosyn inhibit the production of the inflammatory prostaglandin E_2 (PGE_2). This helps to decrease inflammation, decrease scarring and adhesions, and decrease pain.
- Danazol, a testosterone derivative, causes the endometrial implants to shrink by inhibiting gonadotropin release from the hypothalamus; and, subsequently, follicle-stimulating hormone (FSH) and luteinizing hormone (LH) release from the pituitary.
- Lupron and Nafarelin are gonadotropin hormone–releasing agonists, which create a low-estrogen (menopausal) state, resulting in decreased symptoms.

Procedures

Surgery. Scenarios that might warrant surgery include infertility or severe pain. If fertility is desired, removal of the implants will occur typically at the time of laparoscopy. The implants are destroyed by either laser or electrocautery. Laser surgery to restore fertility is successful in about 50% of cases. A total hysterectomy occurs in cases where fertility is not a concern and the scars from endometriosis are extensive.

To prevent premature menopause, it is recommended that the ovaries be preserved whenever possible.

Nonallopathic Treatments

Vaginal depletion packs (vag packs) are small suppositories containing vitamins, minerals, and herbs that are placed deep in the vagina, close to the cervix. They function to

- Improve circulation of the pelvic organs by suspending the uterus higher in the pelvis
- Draw fluid and infectious exudates out of the uterus
- Inhibit local bacterial growth
- Stimulate the body to slough off abnormal cervical cells
- Promote lymphatic drainage

Vitamins, Minerals, and Herbs

- To inhibit the production of the inflammatory prostaglandin E_2 (PGE_2) in favor of the anti-inflammatory prostaglandin E_1 (PGE_1):
  - L-carnitine–750 mg/day
  - Gamma Linolenic Acid (GLA)–240 mg/day
  - Eicosapentaenoic acid/docosahexaenoic acid (EPA/DHA)–750 mg/day
  - Vitamin C–5000 mg/day
  - Pyridoxine–5000 mg/day
- To enhance liver function
  - Methionine–1000 mg/day
  - Choline–1950 mg/day
  - Inositol–650 mg/day
- Milk thistle *(Silybum marianum)* promotes healthy liver function.

16

Female Athlete Triad

WHAT IS IT?

The female athlete triad consists of disordered eating (anorexia nervosa and bulimia nervosa), amenorrhea (primary amenorrhea, secondary amenorrhea, and oligomenorrhea), and osteoporosis.

Anorexia Nervosa and Bulimia Nervosa

Anorexia nervosa
- Refusal to maintain body weight
- Body weight less than 85% of expected
- Intense fear of gaining weight
- Failure to make expected weight gain during period of growth and an individual who denies seriousness of low body weight

Bulimia nervosa
- Recurrent episodes of binge eating
- Lack of control over eating
- Eating excessive amounts during a discrete time period
- Recurrent compensatory behavior, including self-induced vomiting; misuse of laxatives, enemas, or diuretics; and excessive exercise
- Self-evaluation is heavily influenced by body shape and weight, and behavior occurs at least twice a week over several months

Amenorrhea

Alterations of the rhythmic secretions of gonadotropin-releasing hormone (GnRH) (possibly attributable to excessive exercise and other compensatory behaviors) can lead to decreased levels of follicle-stimulating hormone (FSH) and luteinizing hormone

(LH) and, subsequently, to decreased levels of estrogen and progesterone, resulting in amenorrhea.

- Primary amenorrhea
  - The absence of spontaneous uterine bleeding by age 14 without development of secondary sexual characteristics or the absence of spontaneous uterine bleeding by age 16 with otherwise normal development
- Secondary amenorrhea
  - Six-month absence of menstrual bleeding in a woman with regular menses or 12-month absence of menstrual bleeding in a woman with previous oligomenorrhea
  - Oligomenorrhea
  - Infrequent menses

Osteoporosis

Osteoporosis is defined as a decline in bone mass (*osteo*–bone, *porous*–passage, *osis*–condition).

A primary function of estrogen is to inhibit osteoclastic activity. As a result of the hypoestrogenic state, osteoclast-mediated bone resorption is uninhibited, resulting in osteoporosis.

WHO GETS IT?

The female athlete triad historically has been associated with athletes; however, it is now known that the condition is not limited to athletes and may be found commonly among age-matched females.

Technical Note

With the passage of Title IX of the educational assistance act in 1972, any college that accepts federal funding must provide equal opportunities for women and men to participate in athletic programs. As a result, more women and girls are participating in competitive sports. Although many health benefits are associated with sports, problems arise from misuse and overzealousness. Between 15% and 62% of female college athletes have reported disordered eating, and as many as 66% of female athletes have reported amenorrhea.

ETIOLOGY

- Sports and activities that emphasize lean physique or a specific body weight such as gymnastics, figure skating, ballet, distance running, diving, and swimming
- Mental and psychosocial issues such as low self-esteem
- Parents and coaches who place undue expectations on the athlete
- Heavy energy expenditure
- Misinformation about nutrition
- Societal pressure to be thin
- Physical, sexual, or substance abuse

SIGNS AND SYMPTOMS

- Recurrent stress fractures
- Amenorrhea or oligomenorrhea
- Erosion of the tooth enamel from gastric acids produced with recurrent vomiting
- Very thin girl or woman
- Muscle injury
- Parotid swelling as a result of frequent stimulation of the salivary glands from recurrent vomiting
- Tooth marks on the back of the hand from induced vomiting
- Fatigue and decreased ability to concentrate
- Presence of lanugo hair
- Sensitivity to cold
- Heart irregularities
- Chest pain
- Endothelial dysfunction
- Reduced cardiovascular dilation response to exercise
- Increased risk of cardiovascular disease
- Urinary incontinence
- Binge eating
- Eating alone
- Frequent trips to the bathroom during and after meals

DIAGNOSIS

- Comprehensive history and examination

Menstrual History

A history of amenorrhea often is the first sign. However, it is important to remember that amenorrhea has many possible causes.

- Delayed onset of menarche
- History of oligomenorrhea
- Absence of physical signs of ovulation such as mittelschmerz
- Previous or current use of hormonal therapy

Diet History

- It is less threatening to inquire about past disordered eating rather than current.
- What was eaten during the last 24 hours?
- Is the list of "forbidden foods" extensive?
- Happiness with current weight.
- Ideal weight according to patient and highest/lowest weight since menarche.
- Use of diet pills or laxatives.

Exercise History

- Exercise patterns
- Training intensity
- History of previous fractures
- History of overuse injuries

Additional Examination Protocols

- Height
- Weight
- Body mass index (BMI)
- Sexual maturity rating
- Scoliosis
- Neglect/abuse screening
- Blood pressure
- Ultrasound blood flow studies
- Bone Mineral Density (BMD)

Laboratory Tests

- Anemia, especially iron deficiency anemia
- Serum electrolytes
- Enzymes such as amylase and lipase

MANAGEMENT

The primary health care provider needs to be astute and willing to work collaboratively with a multidisciplinary team, including psychologists, dietitians, coaches, teachers, and parents.

- Dietitians facilitate the design of healthy nutritional choices and attaining and maintaining ideal weight. They also can educate regarding prevention of caloric deficit and maintaining positive energy balance.
- Psychiatrists/psychologists manage the eating disorders and esteem concerns.
- Coaches modify exercise intensity. Typically, a 10% to 20% decrease in exercise intensity is needed.
- Teachers and parents monitor progress, assess for compliance, and provide support and encouragement.

Clinical Pearl
Close monitoring of the menstrual status is essential.

Diet

- High-phosphate substances such as artificially carbonated beverages tend to increase bone loss of calcium and should be avoided.
- Red meats should be eaten sparingly because the uric acid from protein synthesis can increase calcium loss.
- High-protein diets cause larger than normal calcium excretion, thereby increasing the potential for bone loss.

Vitamin and Mineral Supplementation

- Daily calcium intake of a minimum 800 mg/day and as much as 1500 mg/day of elemental calcium to prevent osteoporosis

Technical Note

Studies conducted on female athletes with osteoporosis demonstrated a lack of improvement in bone density with calcium supplementation in the presence of amenorrhea. Bone density improved with calcium supplementation only with the return of menses or the addition of estrogen therapy.

- Boron 1 mg a day to aid utilization of calcium
- Vitamin D 800 to 1000 units/day to aid calcium absorption
- Vitamin C up to 2 g/day in split doses can aid development of the collagen portion of bone
- Folic acid

Medications

Birth control or estrogen supplementation often is necessary, especially if a progesterone challenge does not result in the onset of menses.

17

Fibroids

WHAT IS IT?

Fibroids are noncancerous tumors of the uterus that vary in size from very small (the size of an apple seed) to larger than a grapefruit (Figure 17-1).

WHO GETS IT?

Women during their reproductive years. Symptoms of fibroids often begin during the early to middle thirties; however, evidence suggests that fibroids may be present but asymptomatic as early as the middle twenties. Women who are overweight are at higher risk.

ETIOLOGY

Heredity

There is evidence that fibroids are familial.

Estrogen/Progesterone Imbalances

Fibroids are dependent on estrogen for growth; that is, they increase in size and number when the estrogen load is high, such as during pregnancy, with the use of high-estrogen birth control pills, and in insulin resistance. Fibroids shrink when estrogen levels decline, such as in menopause or with the use of progesterone-only birth control methods.

SIGNS AND SYMPTOMS

- A feeling of hardness in the lower abdomen or pelvic area
- Frequent urination

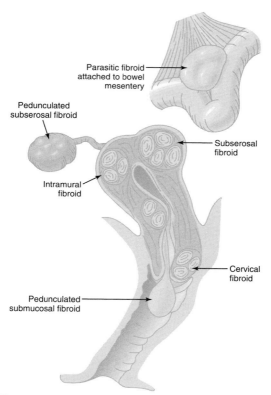

FIGURE 17-1 Uterine fibroids in various anatomic locations. (From Hacker NF, Moore JG, Gambone JC: *Essentials of obstetrics and gynecology,* ed 4, Philadelphia, 2004, WB Saunders.)

- Menorrhagia
- Anemia as a result of months (sometimes years) of menorrhagia
- Blood clots associated with menses
- Hemorrhage
- Dysmenorrhea
- Dyspareunia
- Mittelschmerz (pain at ovulation)
- Reproductive problems, such as miscarriage and infertility
- Low back pain

- Many women who have fibroids frequently have associated symptoms of thinning hair or male balding hair patterns
- Many women with fibroids are asymptomatic

DIAGNOSIS

- Uterus appears enlarged and lumpy on routine pelvic examination
- Pelvic ultrasound
- Magnetic resonance imaging (MRI)
- Computed tomography (CT)
- Laparoscopy
- Hysteroscopy
- Hysterosalpingogram (HSG), x-ray of the uterus with contrast; submucous, interstitial, and subserous may be visualized on HSG
- Dilation and curettage
  Definitive diagnosis of fibroids is by ultrasound of the uterus.

MANAGEMENT

Management is based on factors such as symptoms, age, desire for pregnancy, and size and location of fibroids.

Lifestyle

- Dietary protocol to manage for insulin resistance includes increasing complex carbohydrates and decreasing refined sugars and simple carbohydrates. Insulin resistance can elevate estrogen, which can worsen the symptoms of fibroids. Insulin resistance can occur under conditions of prolonged stress.
- Eliminate caffeine.
- Increase dietary fiber. Whole grains in the form of oats, rice, buckwheat, and millet are excellent sources. They enhance the function of the elimination pathways and provide B vitamins, which are useful in the body's synthesis of the anti-inflammatory prostaglandins.
- Avoid meats, dairy, and poultry from hormone-fattened livestock. These are exogenous sources of estrogens. Red meats and dairy increase systemic production of arachidonic acid, a precursor to the inflammatory prostaglandins.

- Increase intake of all phytoestrogens, particularly the cruciferous vegetables kale, collard greens, cauliflower, cabbage, broccoli, and brussels sprouts, which are sources of calcium and indole-3-carbinol (a necessary precursor in the synthesis of the weaker 2-OH estrogens). Increase intake of legumes, including lentils, chickpeas, and mung beans, and soy products, such as tofu, tempeh, and other soybeans.
- Fruits such as kiwi, figs, raspberries, and oranges are useful adjuncts in the management of fibroids because they are sources of calcium, magnesium, and potassium, which help to relax the muscles and decrease menstrual pain and cramping.

Psychosocial Factors

Stress causes a rise in cortisol, which affects other hormones such as estrogen. Attending to psychosocial stressors is essential to the management of fibroids.

Acupressure

Apply gentle, direct pressure over acupressure points for general reproductive health as follows: spleen 6, located about three to four finger widths above the medial malleolus; hoku hand point at the junction of the thumb and index finger.

Acupuncture

Acupuncture may relieve pain and pelvic congestion. Ren (zhen) 4 is midway between the navel and pubic bone, and du 4 is directly over L2. In traditional Chinese medicine (TCM), these points would be treated concurrently with moxibustion, a warm heat source from burning herbs or needling.

Spinal Manipulation

The nerves that supply the uterus and ovaries exit the spinal cord between the twelfth thoracic and fifth lumbar vertebrae. Spinal assessment and manipulation, which ensures the proper alignment of the vertebrae that protect the spine at these levels and that balance the pelvis, is recommended to alleviate biomechanical distortions and decrease nerve interference.

Massage/Myofascial Release

Some of the pain associated with fibroids can be relieved with low back and abdominal massage.

Medications

Medications such as the gonadotropin-hormone–releasing agonists Lupron and Nafarelin create a low-estrogen (menopausal) state.

Vitamins, Minerals, and Herbs

- Indole-3-carbinol and di-indolylmethane, phytonutrients found in the cruciferous vegetables, help the liver and gut to metabolize for the less potent 2-hydroxy estrogen derivatives.
- Green tea polyphenols may impair the deleterious effects of estrogen.
- Calcium D-glucarate prevents the reabsorption of excreted estrogens from the digestive tract.
- To inhibit the production of the inflammatory prostaglandin E_2 (PGE_2) in favor of the antiinflammatory prostaglandin E_1 (PGE_1):
  - L-carnitine–750 mg/day
  - Gamma-linolenic (GLA)–240 mg/day
  - Eicosapentaenoic acid/docosahexaenoic acid (EPA/DHA)–750 mg/day
  - Vitamin C–5000 mg/day
  - Pyridoxine–5000 mg/day
- To enhance liver function:
  - Methionine–1000 mg/day
  - Choline–1950 mg/day
  - Inositol–650 mg/day
- Milk thistle *(Silybum marianum)* promotes healthy liver function.
- Black cohosh extract (1 to 2 mg of 27-deoxyacteine twice daily).

PROCEDURES

- Surgical removal of the fibroid (myomectomy)
- Surgical removal of the uterus and ovaries (hysterectomy)

- Scenarios that might warrant surgery include excessive bleeding, risk of hemorrhage, an inability to determine whether the tumor is benign, or family history of endometrial and other reproductive tract cancers
- Uterine artery embolization—occlusion of the portion of the uterine artery that supplies the fibroid

NONALLOPATHIC TREATMENTS

Vaginal depletion packs (vag packs) are small suppositories containing vitamins, minerals, and herbs that are placed deep in the vagina, close to the cervix. They function to

- Improve circulation of the pelvic organs by suspending the uterus higher in the pelvis
- Draw fluid and infectious exudates out of the uterus
- Inhibit local bacterial growth
- Stimulate the body to slough off abnormal cervical cells
- Promote lymphatic drainage

18

Fibromyalgia

WHAT IS IT?

Fibromyalgia is a common chronic condition characterized by fatigue; widespread pain; and tenderness in muscles, joints, bones, tendons, and other soft tissues. The pain of fibromyalgia is typically bilateral, and occurs in areas above and below the waist.

WHO GETS IT?

Fibromyalgia occurs primarily in women in their late twenties through fifties.

ETIOLOGY

The cause of fibromyalgia syndrome is unknown. Proposed causes include the following:
- Autoimmune dysfunction
- Sleep disorders
- Abnormal central nervous system functioning
- Autoimmune disorders such as lupus
- Rheumatoid arthritis
- Hypothyroidism
- Aluminum toxicity
- Stress
- Repetitive use
- Physical trauma
- Emotional trauma
- History of a bacterial infection

SIGNS AND SYMPTOMS

Widespread pain occurs above and below the waist and on both sides of the body. Pain and tenderness occurs in at least 11 of 18 (i.e., 9 pairs) tender point sites (Figure 18-1):

- Base of the occiput at the insertion of the suboccipital muscles
- Anterior neck at the lower cervical spine from C5–C7
- The midpoint of the upper trapezius muscle
- Supraspinatus muscle near its medial border above the spine of the scapula
- Second rib at the second costochondral junction
- Lateral epicondyles
- Gluteal muscles at the upper outer quadrant of the buttocks

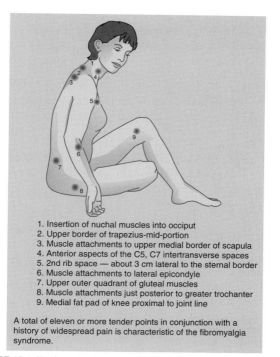

1. Insertion of nuchal muscles into occiput
2. Upper border of trapezius-mid-portion
3. Muscle attachments to upper medial border of scapula
4. Anterior aspects of the C5, C7 intertransverse spaces
5. 2nd rib space — about 3 cm lateral to the sternal border
6. Muscle attachments to lateral epicondyle
7. Upper outer quadrant of gluteal muscles
8. Muscle attachments just posterior to greater trochanter
9. Medial fat pad of knee proximal to joint line

A total of eleven or more tender points in conjunction with a history of widespread pain is characteristic of the fibromyalgia syndrome.

FIGURE 18-1 Tender point sites. (From Goldman L, Ausiello D: *Cecil textbook of medicine,* ed 22, Philadelphia, 2004, WB Saunders.)

- Greater trochanter of the hip
- Medial knee
  Symptoms may worsen in cold or damp weather.
  Associated symptoms include headaches, fatigue, sleep disturbances, morning stiffness, numbness in the hands and feet, anxiety
disorders, facial pain, irritable bowel syndrome, painful menses,
pain between the shoulder blades, skinfold tenderness, dizziness,
mood changes, dry eyes, difficulty concentrating, and depression.

DIAGNOSIS

- It is important to separate true fibromyalgia syndrome from
  the numerous conditions that may manifest with similar
  symptoms, including hypothyroidism, Lyme disease, chronic
  fatigue syndrome, rheumatoid arthritis, vitamin and mineral
  deficiencies, and side effects from medications such as the
  cholesterol-lowering statin drugs.
- The classic fibromyalgia patient has increased sensitivity to
  pain (hyperalgesia) and the perception of pain in response
  to a normally nonpainful stimulus (allodynia).
- The following algorithm proposed by Michael J. Schneider
  can be used to ensure that an accurate diagnosis is made:
  - Blood tests to rule out conditions such as hypothyroidism or
    hyperthyroidism, Graves' disease, and rheumatoid arthritis.
  - Chest x-rays to rule out other pathology.
  - If the patient has a minimum of 3 months of widespread
    pain above and below the waist, on both sides of the body,
    and a minimum of 11 of the 18 identified tender points, a
    diagnosis of fibromyalgia may be made.

MANAGEMENT

Currently, there is no known treatment that benefits all fibromyalgia patients. Patients may need to try several types of modalities to find the one that provides them with the greatest relief
and symptomatic benefit.

- Self-help:
  - Decrease stress.
  - Practice meditation.
  - Assess and modify lifestyle factors that may be affecting the
    condition.

- Avoid temperature extremes.
- Avoid known allergens, processed foods, caffeine, alchohol, and foods manufactured with synthetic hormones or given synthetic hormone injections.
- Nutritional support for the patient with fibromyalgia should be directed toward increasing the anti-inflammatory prostaglandins and decreasing arachidonic acid and the inflammatory prostaglandins. Supporting these processes implies supplementation with the B vitamins, minerals such as magnesium and zinc, phytonutrients such as ginger and curcumin, and the fish oils eicosapentaenoic acid/docosahexaenoic acid (EPA/DHA), and gamma linolenic acid (GLA).
- Malic acid 1200 to 2400 mg/day in divided doses may be of some use in fibromyalgia; however, the evidence remains inconclusive.
  - Malic acid is an alpha-hydroxy organic acid that sometimes is referred to as fruit acid because it is found in apples and other fruits.
  - In a double-blind, placebo-controlled crossover study, subjects with primary fibromyalgia syndrome were randomized to receive a combination of 200 mg of malic acid and 50 mg of magnesium per tablet (three tablets twice a day) or placebo for 4 weeks. This was followed by a 6-month, open-label trial with dose escalating up to six tablets twice a day. Outcome variables were measures of pain and tenderness, as well as functional and psychologic measures.
  - No clear benefit was observed for the malic acid–magnesium combination in the lower-dose blinded trial. But in the open-label trial, at higher doses, there were significant reductions in the severity of all three primary pain/tenderness measures.
- Magnesium 300 to 600 mg/day in divided doses to facilitate the secretion of aluminum. Dietary sources include dairy, fish, leafy greens, soybeans, and molasses.
- Manganese 20 mg/day in divided doses to support thyroid function. Dietary sources include avocados, whole grains, and nuts.
- St. John's wort as prescribed by the treating physician to raise serotonin levels and aid with depression.
- S-adenosyl-L-methionine (SAMe) 1600 mg/day to increase the responsiveness of the cells to serotonin.

- 5-Hydroxytryptophan (5-HTP) 50 to 100 mg three times daily with meals to raise serotonin levels. This should not be used concurrently with selective serotonin reuptake inhibitors (SSRIs) or monoamine oxidase (MAO) inhibitors or other antidepressant medications.

Technical Note

- 5-Hydroxytryptophan (5-HTP) is an intermediary compound produced when the body converts the amino acid tryptophan to serotonin and melatonin. Serotonin is a neurotransmitter that helps the brain's nerve cells to send and receive messages. The sending nerve cell releases serotonin, which is taken up by the receiving nerve cell. In the process, however, some of the serotonin is reabsorbed by an uptake pump. Antidepressants such as Prozac are believed to work by blocking the action of the serotonin uptake pump, thereby increasing the brain's supply of serotonin. Supplements such as 5-HTP are believed to work by increasing the amount of serotonin produced by the brain cells.
- Potential side effects of 5-HTP include nausea and mild digestive disturbances.

Clinical Pearl

Pregnant or nursing women, people with liver or kidney disease, and children with Down syndrome should not use 5-HTP.

Spinal Manipulation

Gentle, low-force spinal manipulation can help to ensure that there are no adverse influences on the nervous system from misaligned spinal vertebrae.

Physical Therapy

- Physical therapies, including postural reeducation, functional exercise training, a supervised progressive cardiovascular exercise

program, core stabilization exercises, electrical muscle stimulation, diaphragmatic breathing, pool therapy, gentle stretching, self-pacing, and hot packs
- Biofeedback
- Cognitive-behavioral pain therapy education regarding chronic pain mechanisms and strategies for management

Exercise

Low-impact exercises such as walking or swimming may be helpful.

Massage Therapy

Massage therapies include skin rolling and trigger point therapy. Caution should be used, because deep tissue massage may result in the condition's flaring up.

Medications

- Analgesics/anti-inflammatories, including nonsteroidal anti-inflammatory drugs (NSAIDs), acetaminophen, tramadol, and gabapentin
- Muscle relaxers
- Benzodiazepines
- Antidepressant drugs such as Prozac

19

Incontinence

Fecal Incontinence

WHAT IS IT?

Fecal incontinence (bowel incontinence) is a loss of control of bowel movements, leakage of stool, and, at the extreme, total loss of bowel control.

WHO GETS IT?

Fecal incontinence occurs in both sexes and in all age groups; however, it is more prevalent in older women.

ETIOLOGY

- Muscle damage:
  - Damage of the muscles of the anal sphincter as a result of a difficult delivery, episiotomy, or use of forceps. The younger woman can compensate; however, as she ages and muscle laxity occurs, the changes in anal sphincter pressure may result in fecal incontinence. Some women notice fecal incontinence immediately after giving birth.
  - Pelvic floor compromise as a result of childbirth.
  - Rectocele as a result of aging.
  - Constipation. Hardened stools become lodged in the rectum, and watery stools leak around the hard stool. The impacted stools cause the muscles of the rectum to stretch and weaken.
- Nerve damage:
  - The nerves that control the anal sphincter and rectum exit the spine at the sacrum and follow a course to the anal sphincter.

- These nerves can be damaged as a result of injury; child-birth; repeated straining to stool; and conditions such as stroke, diabetes, and multiple sclerosis.
- The sensory nerves to the anal sphincter also can become damaged, and, as a result, the individual loses the sensation of stools in the rectum.
- Rectal storage capacity. Conditions such as irritable bowel syndrome can cause irritation and scarring, which impairs the ability of the rectum to stretch. As a result, rectal volume is compromised.
- Diarrhea. Looser stools are more difficult to control.

SIGNS AND SYMPTOMS

- Urgency
- Loss of bowel control

DIAGNOSIS

- Signs and symptoms
- History
- Physical examination, including a digital rectal examination
- Additional diagnostic tests, such as
  - Anal manometry, which assesses the integrity of the anal sphincter and rectum
  - Anorectal ultrasound
  - Proctography (defecography), which shows how much stool the rectum can hold, how well the rectum holds it, and how well the rectum can evacuate the stool
  - Anal electromyography (EMG), which evaluates for nerve damage often associated with obstetric injury
  - Proctosigmoidoscopy to evaluate for inflammation, tumors, scar tissue, and other disease processes

MANAGEMENT

- Self-help

Diet

- Identify food triggers by keeping a food diary. Common triggers include caffeine, dairy products, alcohol, spicy foods, pork byproducts, sweeteners, fatty foods, and some fruits.

- Eat smaller meals.
- Do not drink fluids with meals.
- Keep well hydrated.
- Modulate fiber intake. Depending on whether constipation or diarrhea is the cause of the incontinence, it may take a course of trial and error to determine the right amount of fiber. Soluble-fiber foods such as bananas, smooth peanut butter, oatmeal, yogurt, and rice are recommended in most cases over insoluble-fiber foods, which slow gastric transit time.

Physical Therapy

- Bowel training. The patient is trained to empty the bowels at a specific time of day. In addition, the patient relearns how to control the bowels and strengthen the involved muscles. Biofeedback and pelvic floor exercises typically are included.
- Biofeedback to strengthen and coordinate the pelvic floor muscles. Biofeedback is coordinated with pelvic floor (Kegel) exercises.
- Pelvic floor (Kegel) exercises (see Appendix).

Acupuncture

Acupuncture and herb treatments are often targeted at correcting "sinking" spleen deficiency and spleen and kidney yang deficiency.

Spinal Manipulation

Spinal manipulation is performed to influence the sacral nerves.

Medications

Depending on the cause, bulk laxatives, stool softeners, antidiarrheal drugs such as loperamide (Imodium), and medications used for irritable bowel syndrome (IBS) are administered.

Procedures

- Sacral nerve stimulation via a pulse generator (see Appendix)
- Surgical recommendations depend on the cause and severity of the condition and response to other modes of treatment; these include the following.

- Colostomy for severe conditions
- Sphincteroplasty to repair a weakened anal sphincter
- Procedures to manage for rectal prolapse

Urinary Incontinence

WHAT IS IT?

Urinary incontinence is the inability to control urine flow.

Technical Note

Categories of urinary incontinence include the following: stress incontinence, which occurs as a result of pressure on the bladder from lifestyle factors such as exercise, pregnancy, laughing, or coughing; urge incontinence, the inability to sustain control over the urge to urinate, frequently seen postpartum and in people with conditions such as diabetes, stroke, or multiple sclerosis; overflow incontinence, which can occur as a result of conditions such as diabetes and spinal cord injury, but more commonly is seen in men as a result of an enlarged prostate; and functional incontinence, which primarily occurs in the elderly as a result of degenerative and other aging disorders that slow movement.

WHO GETS IT?

Men and women of all ages. Many women report incontinence during pregnancy and postpartum.

Clinical Pearl

Urinary incontinence often goes unreported for years because many women are either embarrassed by the condition or believe there is no cure.

ETIOLOGY

- Pelvic floor compromise as a result of childbirth.
- Nerve damage:
  - The nerves that control the bladder exit the spine at the sacrum.

- These nerves can be damaged as a result of injury, childbirth, stroke, multiple sclerosis, and diabetes.
- Bladder storage capacity. Conditions such as irritable bowel syndrome (IBS) can cause irritation and scarring, which can affect the bladder.
- Urinary tract infections (UTIs).

SIGNS AND SYMPTOMS

- Urinary frequency
- Urinary urgency
- Stress incontinence
- Complete loss of bladder control

DIAGNOSIS

- Careful history
- Signs and symptoms
- Urinalysis and blood tests to rule out UTI
- Cystoscopy
- Pelvic/abdominal ultrasound
- Contrast studies of the kidneys and bladder
- EMG
- Urinary stress tests, which check for urine loss while performing functions such as exercise or coughing
- Urinary postvoid residual, which assesses the amount of urine that remains in the bladder after urination
- Pad test, which uses the weight of a saturated sanitary pad after exercise to evaluate degree of urine loss

MANAGEMENT

Lifestyle Management

- Diet—avoid known triggers such as caffeine and alcohol
- Keep a daily food/symptom diary to identify other potential triggers
- Bladder training
- Timed voiding—urinating according to an identified schedule every day
- Pelvic floor (Kegel) exercises with or without vaginal cones (see Appendix)

- Pessaries and bladder neck support devices may be used to manage for prolapse
- Urethral opening occlusion devices such as tampons, Reliance, CapSure, and FemAssist

Physical Therapy

- Bladder training/timed voiding. The patient is trained to empty the bladder at a specific time of day. In addition, the patient relearns how to control the bladder and strengthen the involved muscles. Biofeedback and pelvic floor exercises typically are included.
- Biofeedback to strengthen and coordinate the pelvic floor muscles. Biofeedback is coordinated with pelvic floor (Kegel) exercises.
- Pelvic floor (Kegel) exercises (see Appendix).
- Pelvic floor stimulation (InterStim therapy). Electrical therapies are applied directly over the pelvic floor muscles.

Spinal Manipulation

Spinal manipulation is performed to stimulate the sacral nerves.

MEDICATIONS

- Tolterodine (Detrol)
- Tolterodine extended release (Detrol LA)
- Trospium CHLORIDE (Sanctura)
- Oxybutynin patch (Oxytrol) for overactive bladder
- Antibiotics if bacterial infection is identified as a cause

PROCEDURES

- Sacral nerve stimulation by direct placement of a pulse generator after testing confirms treatment efficacy (see Appendix).
- Periurethral bulking injections. Collagen injections into the tissue around the urethra adds bulk and retards leakage. More than one treatment typically is required.
- Botulinum toxin (Botox) sometimes is injected into the bladder muscles to relieve muscle spasms. It can provide symptom relief for up to 1 year.

SURGERY

- Pubovaginal, tension-free vaginal tape (TVT) and other sling procedures
- Burch urethropexy procedures

20

Infections

Primary Infections of the Vulva

WHAT IS IT?

The term *vulva infection* is used to describe inflammation/infection of the area of the genital tract that is bordered by the labia majora and includes the labia, clitoris, and vaginal opening.

Infections of the vulvar typically begin as an irritation or inflammation and become infected from scratching.

WHO GETS IT?

Women of any age may get an infection of the vulva.

ETIOLOGY

Can begin as allergic irritations from the use of vaginal sprays, scented toilet paper, soaps, feminine deodorants, and douches and is compounded by conditions such as postmenopausal dryness/atrophy and diabetes.

Drug reactions may occur in the presence of atrophic tissue.

True vulva infections are most commonly secondary to vaginal infections and are caused by any or all of the pathogens that cause vaginal infections, including *Mycoplasma, Trichomonas vaginalis,* herpes simplex, *Candida, Neisseria gonorrhoeae,* and *Chlamydia trachomatis.*

SIGNS AND SYMPTOMS

- Itching, which leads to scratching, which can aggravate the infection and cause a secondary infection

- Swelling
- Redness
- Oozing
- Crusting
- Scaling
- Vesicles, which may break, pus, crust, and scale
- Other signs and symptoms associated with vaginal infections (see section on vaginal infections)

DIAGNOSIS

- Detailed and accurate history, which should elicit the causative factors
- Signs and symptoms
- Culture
- Wet mount

MANAGEMENT
Medical

- Cortisone creams for the irritation and antibacterial/antifungal agents as warranted by the identified causative pathogen

Manipulation

- Ensure that the pelvis and spinal structures are functioning optimally

Ancillary/Concurrent Lifestyle Factors

- Eliminate the causative factor: discontinue the use of any soaps, powders, deodorants, toilet paper, or other products that may be correlated directly with the onset of the irritation/infection.
- Keep the area cool and dry.
- Wear cotton undergarments to allow for adequate ventilation of the area.
- Apply calamine lotion.
- Oatmeal baths such as the Aveeno colloidal may be useful.
- Aloe vera compresses may be helpful.
- Cold compresses of natural yogurt can be used to relieve the itching.

Vaginal Infections

GENERAL CONSIDERATIONS

The pH of the vaginal tract normally is slightly acidic (3.8 to 4.2). Factors that create a shift in the pH predispose to vaginal infections. These include the following:

- Douching
- Diabetes
- Antibiotics
- Hormonal birth control methods such as oral contraceptives
- Decreased immunity
- Pregnancy

Technical Note

Local endogenous flora such as *Lactobacillus* maintain the acidic environment of the vagina by converting sugars to lactic acid. Antibiotics and douching interfere with this process by destroying the endogenous bacteria. Systemic conditions such as diabetes in turn play a role by altering the sugar content of the cells. For this reason, dietary habits and insulin resistance inadvertently contribute to vaginal infections.

CANDIDIASIS (YEAST INFECTIONS)

What Is It?

Candidiasis is infection caused by the fungi *Candida albicans, Candida tropicalis,* and *Candida glabrata. Candida* is part of the normal endogenous flora. Infection is due to systemic and local overgrowth.

   Candida is not a sexually transmitted disease (STD); however, in refractory cases, treatment of the partner may be needed.

Who Gets It?

All women. Some estimates suggest that 75% of women will have an episode of candidiasis at least once, and 40% will have recurrent infections.

Etiology

- Alterations in the vaginal milieu as a result of predisposing factors such as

- Pregnancy
- Systemic antibiotics
- High-estrogen oral contraceptives
- Use of corticosteroids
- Decreased immunity as seen in acquired immunodeficiency syndrome (AIDS), premature infants, and patients on chemotherapy or radiation therapy
- Diabetes
- Frequent douching
- Improper sanitary habits such as wiping from the back to the front following bowel movements

Signs and Symptoms

The presence of vaginal discharge that is white, has a curdlike/cottage cheese appearance, and adheres to the vaginal wall; attempts to remove the white "coating" may leave a hemorrhagic area.
- Intense pruritus (severe itching)
- Dysuria (pain with urination)
- Dyspareunia (pain with intercourse)
- Burning or inflammation of the vulvar and vaginal surfaces
   The classic presentation is vulvovaginitis and intense pruritus accompanied by whitish discharge.

Diagnosis

- Symptoms. Vaginal discharge is white, thick, and cottage cheese–like in appearance, and adheres to the vaginal surface.
- Wet mount preparation. The discharge is mixed with 10% potassium hydroxide (KOH) or saline solution in order to lyse the white and red blood cells and epithelial cells. The hyphae, pseudohyphae, or budding yeast cells are viewed under a microscope.
- Fungal cultures may be used in recurrent or resistant cases.

Management

Lifestyle factors

- The vaginal area should be kept clean and ventilated. This might necessitate sleeping without underwear, avoiding tight clothing, wearing skirts instead of pants, and wearing undergarments made of natural fibers such as cotton.

- It has been suggested that *Candida* may survive normal wash and dry cycles. Undergarments should be prewashed, washed in bleach or boiling water, ironed, or replaced.
- To avoid reinnoculation from the anus to the vagina, patients should be advised to wipe from front to back after bowel movements.
- Douche with vinegar water, 1/2 cup vinegar in a shallow tub.
- Take sitz baths, 1/2 cup salt or 1/2 cup vinegar in a shallow tub.
- Avoid douching during menses.
- Avoid douching purely for feminine hygiene purposes because this changes the pH of the vagina and can set up an environment for other vaginal infections.
- Avoid intercourse while infection is active.
- Urinate before and after intercourse.
- Avoid use of spermicides and other potential irritants.
- Use condoms.
- Avoid chemical irritants such as colored or scented toilet paper, feminine deodorant sprays, and scented tampons or pads.
- Use pads at night instead of tampons.
- Garlic clove suppositories may be helpful.
- Gentian violet may be applied topically for resistant strains. A maximum of three applications can be used either once per week for 4 weeks or monthly after menses for 4 months. Gentian violet is derived from the dried root of the *Gentiana lutea* plant.
- Get adequate rest.

Diet
- Avoid drugs, caffeine, and cigarette smoke.
- Avoid fermented beverages, including wine, beer, root beer, and cider.
- Avoid allergenic foods, which include fungi such as mushrooms, and foods that contain yeasts such as some breads and cheeses.
- Drink pure, unsweetened cranberry juice.
- Avoid sugars, artificial sweeteners, concentrated fruit juices, and doughnuts.
- Boost the immune system with a healthy diet, including immune-supporting vitamins such as B_2, B_5, and C, food sources of which include whole grains, eggs, fish, poultry, spinach and other vegetables, and citrus fruits and berries; vitamin A, food sources of which include brightly colored fruits and vegetables; vitamin E, found in nuts and wheat

germ; and the minerals selenium, found in nuts and whole grains, and zinc, found in large quantities in eggs, seafood, whole grains, and legumes.

Supplements

- Probiotics. Supplementation with live *Lactobacillus acidophilus* cultures and UltraBifidus. Alternatively, four to six acidophilus capsules can be inserted into the vagina 2 to 3 days before menses.
- Supplementation with caprylic acid (Capristatin), a naturally occurring nystatin.
- Ingesting natural, no-sugar yogurt with live cultures of *L. acidophilus.*

Medications

- Over-the-counter vaginal creams such as clotrimazole (Gyne-Lotrimin) 1% 5 g, or miconazole (Monistat) 2% 5 g, typically used at bedtime for 3 or 7 days.
- Prescription medications such as terconazole 0.4% 5 g, 7-day vaginal cream; terconazole 80 mg, 3-day suppository; and miconazole 1200 mg single-dose treatment.
- Oral medications also are available, including one-dose fluconazole 150 mg and 3-day itraconazole 200 mg.
- Resistant cases may be treated with up to 2 weeks of topical or oral medications followed by suppressive therapy with clotrimazole 500 mg vaginal suppository or fluconazole 100 mg orally once weekly.

BACTERIAL VAGINOSIS

What Is It?

Bacterial vaginosis is a condition in which the normal balance of bacteria in the vagina is disrupted and overgrowth of certain bacteria occurs. Bacterial vaginosis can be transmitted sexually and is considered an STD; however, it also can occur in the absence of sexual contact.

Who Gets It?

Primarily women who are sexually active. It is the most frequently diagnosed symptomatic vaginitis in American women.

Etiology

- Previously called *Haemophilus* vaginitis, nonspecific vaginitis, and *Corynebacterium vaginale,* bacterial vaginosis is a symbiotic infection in the vaginal tract caused by abnormal proliferation of *Gardnerella vaginalis* and microbes such as *Bacteroides, Prevotella, Peptococcus (Peptostreptococcus), Mobiluncus,* and *Mycoplasma hominis.*
- Risk factors for bacterial vaginosis include having multiple sex partners or a new sexual relationship, repeated douching, oral-genital sexual activity, previous history of STDs, use of the intrauterine device (IUD), and pregnancy.

Signs and Symptoms

- Burning and itching of the external genitalia may be present.
- Vaginal discharge that is profuse, grayish or white, and foul smelling, and that may have a fishy odor that is worse after intercourse.

Diagnosis

- By signs and symptoms
- Wet mount preparation and microscopic examination; "clue cells" (vaginal epithelium and adherent bacteria) are observed along with clumps of bacteria
- Vaginal pH greater than 4.5
- Positive amine "whiff" test when KOH is applied to the vaginal secretions

Management

Medications

- Oral metronidazole 500 mg twice daily for 7 days has a 90% to 95% cure rate; 2 g orally as a single dose does not have as high a cure rate.
- Oral clindamycin 300 mg for 7 days has a 90% cure rate.
- Vaginal metronidazole gel for 5 days or clindamycin cream for 7 days.
- In pregnancy, it is advised to use only vaginal metronidazole during the first trimester because vaginal clindamycin appears to increase the rate of preterm delivery. After the first trimester, medical doctors may prescribe oral metronidazole or clindamycin.

Technical Note

Bacterial vaginosis in pregnancy has been associated with preterm labor, premature rupture of membranes, and infection of the amniotic fluid.

- The Centers for Disease Control and Prevention (CDC) does not recommend treating male sexual partners. Although it is recognized that 90% of male sexual partners of women with bacterial vaginosis also culture positive for *Gardnerella* vaginosis, treatment of male partners does not appear to reduce the rate of recurrence. Condom use does reduce the rate of recurrence. Female sex partners should be treated.
- Bacterial vaginosis sometimes will clear up without treatment; however, generally it is recommended that all women with symptoms of bacterial vaginosis should be treated to avoid complications such as pelvic inflammatory disease (PID).

Adjunctive management
- Drinking pure, unsweetened cranberry juice
- Vinegar/water douches, 5 tablespoons to 2 quarts of water
- Garlic suppositories; the clove is crushed, wrapped in gauze, and inserted as a tampon; may cause mild vaginal stinging
- Goldenseal myrrh douche, 1 tablespoon goldenseal to 3 cups of hot water, simmered, strained, and cooled
- Condoms
- Abstinence
- Boosting the immune system with vitamins, minerals, and adequate rest
- In some cases, treating the partner may be recommended

TRICHOMONAS VAGINITIS
What Is It?

Trichomonas vaginitis is an STD caused by the flagellated protozoan *Trichomonas vaginalis*.

Who Gets It?

Sexually active women of reproductive age

Etiology

Infection by *T. vaginalis*. *Trichomonas* does not survive in the normally low acidic pH of the vaginal vault. However, with a shift in the pH as occurs during menses, times of stress, and in the presence of other organisms such as streptococci, infection may occur.

Signs and Symptoms

Signs and symptoms frequently occur after menses and include the following:
- Vaginal discharge that is profuse; malodorous; yellowish, green, or grey in color; and frothy or bubbly
- Red and sore vaginal opening
- Itching and burning
- Dysuria
- Dyspareunia
- Strawberry appearance of the cervix in approximately 10% of cases

  In extreme cases, the entire vulvar area, the inside of the thighs, and the anus may be affected.

Diagnosis

Diagnosis is by signs and symptoms and by microscopic examination of the vaginal discharge, which demonstrates the presence of the protozoan and excessive white blood cells. When warmed to body temperature, active movement of the protozoan may be apparent. The vaginal pH is greater than 5.

Management

Medications
- Single, oral 2 g dose of metronidazole has a 98% cure rate.
- If infection occurs during the first trimester of pregnancy, clotrimazole 100 mg vaginal tablets are used for 2 weeks for symptomatic relief.

Adjunctive management
- Treat the sexual partner.
- Use condoms.
- Vinegar douche, 5 tablespoons to 2 quarts of water, to acidify the environment.

- Chickweed douche, 3 tablespoons of chickweed to 1 quart of water. Cover and let sit for 5 to 10 minutes; strain. Douche daily for 1 week.
- Garlic suppositories should be replaced every 12 hours.
- Goldenseal-myrrh douche.
- Keep the vulvar area dry.

POSTMENOPAUSAL BLADDER INFECTIONS

Studies suggest that as many as 40% of postmenopausal women with a diagnosis of urinary tract infection do not have bacteria in the urine. When present, the bacteria most commonly identified is *Escherichia coli.*

Signs and Symptoms

- Burning pain on urination
- Increased urinary frequency and urgency
- Turbid, foul-smelling urine
- Lower abdominal pain

Prevention

- Enhance urine flow by drinking lots of water.
- Avoid soft drinks and concentrated fruit drinks.
- Pure cranberry and blueberry juices help prevent bacterial adherence to the endothelial cells of the bladder.

Management

- Drink copious quantities of fluids, including water, pure, unsweetened blueberry and cranberry juices, and goldenseal tea
- Urinate after intercourse
- Eliminate food allergens
- Antibiotics if an identified pathogen is present

Clinical Pearl

When antibiotics are used, supplementation with probiotics such as L. acidophilus *is necessary to restore normal digestive flora.*

HERPES

What Is It?

- Infection of the vulva and cervix by herpes simplex virus.
- Herpes simplex virus is an enveloped, deoxyribonucleic acid (DNA)–containing virus that is subgrouped into two varieties. Herpes simplex virus 1 (HSV-1) usually is associated with oronasal infections (i.e., cold sores), and herpes simplex virus 2 (HSV-2) usually causes infections of the vulva, vagina, cervix, and anus. Either type may be found in either location of the body.
- Herpes simplex virus is a highly contagious STD. The infected partner may or may not have active lesions and may be asymptomatic yet actively shedding viral particles before the outbreak of the vesicle. Many individuals describe a prodromal phase of malaise, fever, tingling of the vulvar skin, and inguinal adenopathy before the outbreak of a vesicle. Following infection, the incubation period is 2 to 7 days before the onset of a primary herpes infection. Vesicles develop on the vulva and rupture after several days, leaving shallow ulcers, which often are painful.
- During the primary infection, the ulcers persist for 1 to 2 weeks and then heal spontaneously. The ulcers may develop a secondary bacterial infection. This causes more pain and delays healing. Viral shedding may persist for 2 to 3 weeks after complete resolution of the lesions.
- The genital herpes virus is latent and resides in the dorsal root ganglion S2, S3, S4 and within the autonomic nerves along the uterosacral ligaments.
- Recurrences appear to be associated with stress, emotional upheaval, and immunosuppressive states. Symptoms of recurrent infection usually are milder.
- Complications:
  - HSV-2 has been associated with the development of severe dysplasia and invasive cervical carcinoma.
  - HSV-2 infection during pregnancy increases the risk of neonatal infection and neurologic injury, with significant fetal morbidity and mortality rates. During early pregnancy, HSV-2 infection increases the risk for spontaneous abortion.

Who Gets It?

- Any sexually active female

Etiology

- Infection by the herpes simplex virus

Signs and Symptoms

- Small blisters at the site of infection 3 to 4 days following the infection
- Lesions may tingle, itch, burn, break, ooze, or scab over
- Abnormal bleeding
- Vaginal pain
- Dysuria
- Dyspareunia
- Leukorrhea
- Inguinal adenopathy
- Concurrent symptoms include fever, malaise, headache, myalgia, and diffuse low back pain
- Urethral or vaginal discharge may occur

Diagnosis

- By signs and symptoms
- Viral inclusion bodies (giant cells) recognized on cytologic (Papanicolaou [Pap]) smear
- Herpes simplex virus culture ideally obtained from the vesicles, rather than the crusted ulcers
- Serologic tests for viral type antibodies may be used to determine past exposure

Management

There is no known cure for herpes. Management is directed at symptomatic relief and shortening the period of the outbreak.

Lifestyle

- Regular Pap smears
- Decrease stress
- Cold compresses of Burow's solution

- Sitz baths
- Ease the pain of urination by directing the stream away from the lesions with a rolled tissue, or urinate while pouring warm water over the area

Vitamin and mineral supplementation
- Lysine 800 to 1000 mg/day during the active infection
- Lysine 312 to 400 mg/day for maintenance
- Foods with high lysine content include fish, chicken, beef, eggs, cheese, pork, lamb, mung beans, lima beans, dairy cow and goat milk, cottage cheese, brewer's yeast, shellfish, and soybeans and other beans
- Avoid foods with a high arginine content (e.g., nuts, seeds, carob, and chocolate) because they might encourage viral growth

Medications

Antivirals. Antiviral medications come in varying doses based on first-time outbreak, recurrent outbreak, or suppression.
- Valtrex
- Famvir

Acyclovir (Zovirax) is used to reduce the duration of viral shedding, the time of healing, the duration of symptoms, and the clinical course of the disease.

Oral acyclovir is given as 200 mg tablets five times daily for 5 to 7 days, and reduces the clinical course by approximately 1 week.

The benefits from topical application of acyclovir are unequivocal. Intravenous acyclovir is reserved for patients with severe systemic infections.

Technical Note
Acyclovir must not be used by women who are pregnant or who may become pregnant.

21

Infertility

WHAT IS IT?

- Infertility is the inability to get pregnant after 1 year of regular sexual activity. Primary infertility implies that there is no history of a successful pregnancy. Secondary infertility implies that there has been a previous successful pregnancy.
- For fertility to occur, the man must produce sperm of sufficient quality and motility, otherwise known as the seminal factor; the sperm must be deposited in the cervix; and the woman must produce a healthy ovum, have a healthy uterus, and have patent fallopian tubes.
- Sterility is the absolute inability to ovulate or produce sperm.

WHO GETS IT?

Statistics show that male infertility accounts for approximately 30% to 40% of all infertility, female infertility accounts for approximately 30% to 40% of all infertility, and shared infertility accounts for approximately 20% to 30% of all infertility.

ETIOLOGY

Male Infertility

Factors that decrease sperm quality, quantity, or viability all will impair male fertility. These include the following:
- Chronic illness
- Mumps
- Prostatitis
- Genital diseases

- Anabolic steroid abuse
- Environmental pollution
- Chronic exposure to nicotine and tobacco smoke
- Lack of knowledge about effective sexual technique
- Tight pants, athletic supporters, hot tubs, long hot showers, saunas, and other lifestyle factors that can result in elevated scrotal temperature

Female Infertility

- Anovulation—the eggs are not released.
- Tubal factor—the fallopian tubes are not patent because of scarring from infection, scar tissue from previous medical procedures, or blockage from conditions such as endometriosis. This accounts for approximately 30% of female infertility.
- Inadequate ovulation. Conditions that cause inadequate ovulation include Turner's syndrome, premature menopause or premature ovarian failure, and polycystic ovary syndrome (also known as Stein-Leventhal syndrome). Inadequate ovulation accounts for approximately 30% of female infertility.
- Cervical patency, including a pinhole-size cervical os, thickened cervical mucus that hinders the transport of sperm, and cervical polyps. This accounts for approximately 20% of female infertility.
- Uterine patency (from scarring, a retroverted uterus, endometriosis, or fibroids) accounts for approximately 20% of female infertility.
- Other factors that influence infertility include emotional stress, prolonged contraception, increased age, environmental pollutants, inadequate hormonal function, and misalignment of the spinal vertebrae.

SIGNS AND SYMPTOMS

- Inability to conceive

DIAGNOSIS

Diagnosis for infertility involves one or more of the following procedures.

Female Infertility

Hormonal assessment

- Day 3 follicle-stimulating hormone (FSH). A high level of FSH is a signal that estrogen levels are lower than anticipated, implying that development of the ovarian follicles is inadequate. Healthy follicular development would result in sufficient quantities of estrogen.
- Day 3 luteinizing hormone (LH) to determine the FSH-to-LH ratio. A ratio of greater than 2.5 is an indication of poor ovarian reserve, even in the presence of normal FSH levels. Ovarian reserve is an indication of the quality of the eggs remaining in the woman's ovaries.
- Day 3 estradiol.
- The clomiphene citrate challenge test (CCCT) is used to assess ovarian reserve more accurately. The patient takes 100 mg of Clomid on days 5 to 9, and FSH is measured again on day 10. An elevated day 10 FSH is an indication that there will be a decreased response to injectable FSH in assisted reproductive cycles, which is a cause of low rates of pregnancy success and high rates of miscarriage.
- Thyroid function tests—thyroid-stimulating hormone (TSH), T_3, and T_4. Hypothyroid and hyperthyroid function can cause anovulatory cycles and miscarriage; hyperthyroidism also can be a cause of fetal malformation and premature labor.
- Human chorionic gonadotropin (HCG), produced by the placenta, is an indication of pregnancy.
- The androgens, testosterone and androsterone. Elevated levels can cause anovulatory cycles.
- Hysterosalpingogram (HSG). The HSG allows the uterine cavity and the fallopian tubes to be visualized. It is an x-ray of the uterus following injection of a contrast medium. Patent fallopian tubes permit the contrast material to spill out and be visualized in the abdominal cavity, whereas blocked fallopian tubes will not.
- Rubin test. Carbon dioxide gas is injected into the uterus and tubes. Shoulder pain caused by escaping gas is an indication of patent fallopian tubes. This is a low-cost, low-specificity screening procedure.
- Laparoscopy is a minor surgical procedure whereby the abdominal cavity is distended with carbon dioxide gas.

The incision is made in the navel, and a long scope is inserted through the incision into the abdominal cavity. The patency of the tubes and uterus is visualized clearly.

- Postcoital test (also known as the Sims test or Huhner test). Microscopic evaluation of the cervical mucus, 2 to 6 hours following intercourse and around ovulation. Cervical mucus should be clear, and sperm still should be active. The presence of inactive sperm is an indication of cervical mucus with sperm antibodies.
- Endometrial biopsy. A small sample of the lining of the uterus is excised and viewed under a microscope. Cancerous and other abnormal cells are identified, and the endometrium is evaluated for normal stages of change during the menstrual cycle.

Male Infertility

Assessments for male and female infertility should be performed concurrently and include the following:

- Semen analysis. Ideally, the sample should be obtained following 2 to 3 days of abstinence and evaluated within 1 to 2 hours of collection. The assessment includes the following:
  - Sperm motility, or evaluation of the forward movement of sperm cells, including an assessment of the speed of sperm movement.
  - Sperm agglutination—whether the sperm travel independently or clumped together.
  - Sperm morphology, or how many sperm are normal.
  - Sperm viability, which is the percentage of sperm that appear to be alive. This process is performed with the use of a staining technique.
  - Semen volume, or the amount of fluid that makes up the semen, which is an assessment of total sperm production by the testes.
  - Sperm count/concentration, or the number of sperm in a standard given volume.
  - The presence of white blood cells or other indicators of infection.
  - The presence of varicocele, which potentially obstructs the flow of semen.
- Male hormonal evaluation:

- Hormone analysis, although not routinely warranted, may be recommended and includes assessment of testosterone and FSH or LH levels.
- Antisperm antibodies. A high concentration of antisperm antibodies can interfere with sperm function.

MANAGEMENT

The management of infertility is based on the outcomes of the previously described diagnostic procedures.

Lifestyle

- Modify the diet to include to include intake of whole grains, organic fruits and vegetables, seeds and nuts, and sufficient amounts of water.
- Limit or eliminate tobacco, alcohol, and caffeine.
- Limit refined sugars and processed foods.
- Maintain healthy weight.
- Practice spiritual growth (e.g., prayer and meditation). Studies have shown that prayer and belief in a higher power may enhance fertility.
- Utilize stress reduction techniques.
- Exercise for general health and perform cross-crawl exercises for fertility enhancement. General Nutritional Recommendations for Female Infertility
- Eicosapentaenoic acid/docosahexaenoic acid (EPA/DHA) (2000 to 8000 mg daily) to improve ovulation and uterine function.
- Vitamin B_6 in a complex (100 to 600 mg daily) to increase pituitary activity, support the nervous system, and decrease stress. Food sources include brewer's yeast, brown rice, whole grains, chicken, eggs, and fish.
- Selenium (75 mcg daily). Food source includes brewer's yeast, meats, seafood, brown rice, whole grains, and nuts.
- Vitamin E (200 to 600 IU daily). Food sources include nuts, vegetable oils, and wheat germ.
- Beta-carotene is useful for ovulation.
- Vitamin C may aid in the production of female sex hormones.
- Iron, if anemia is found to be a probable cause of the infertility. Food sources include red meats, green leafy vegetables, whole grains, liver, fish, and eggs.
- Zinc 80 mg/day.

- Herbs such as chaste tree berry *(Vitex)* if hyperprolactinemia is a cause of infertility, black cohosh (RemiFemin), and ginseng, all of which modulate the hormonal milieu.

General Nutritional Recommendations for Male Infertility

- Zinc (80 mg daily and up to 80 mg three times per day) to aid sperm count, vitality, and spermatogenesis. Food sources include eggs, legumes, seafood, whole grains, pork, beef, lamb, chicken (especially the dark meat), and peanut butter.
- Vitamin A (5000 IU daily) as retinal, to aid spermatogenesis. Food sources include watermelon and other brightly colored fruits and vegetables.

Clinical Pearl

Conversion of retinol to retinal may be blocked by alcohol. Alcohol use should be minimized.

- Vitamin C (2000 to 6000 mg daily) for sperm agglutination. Food sources include citrus fruits and berries.
- Vitamin B_6 in a B complex (100 to 600 mg daily) to increase pituitary activity. Food sources include whole grains, eggs, fish, brewer's yeast, brown rice, chicken, and dairy products.
- Vitamin E (200 to 600 IU daily) as an antioxidant. Food sources include nuts, wheat germ, and vegetable oils.
- Selenium (75 mcg) as an antioxidant. Food sources include brewer's yeast, meats, nuts, whole grains, and brown rice.

Massage

- Massage for relaxation and to decrease hypertonicity and trigger points in the pelvic muscles.
- Specific muscle stripping and muscle release techniques should be applied to the adductors and psoas.

Spinal Manipulation

Assessment and correction of misalignments in the spinal vertebrae with emphasis placed on the spinal nerves that provide innervation to the reproductive tract in both the male and female.

Medications

Medications are targeted to the identified cause of infertility and management strategies and include the following:

- Estrogen therapy to induce cervical secretions and to manage for thickened cervical mucus
- Clomid, Serophene, and Pergonal, which mature the ovarian follicles and stimulate ovulation
- Bromocriptine (Parlodel) to treat anovulation caused by elevated prolactin levels
- Low-dose corticosteroids to modulate overproduction of the androgens and to retard sperm antibody production
- HCG or Ovidrel to time ovulation during in vitro fertilization (IVF)
- Progesterone to support the development of the endometrium and to prevent miscarriage, especially during IVF cycles

PROCEDURES

- Laparoscopic tubal surgery if one or both of the fallopian tubes are plugged

Intrauterine Insemination

- Intrauterine insemination (IUI) involves placing sperm directly inside the uterus to increase the chances of fertilization. IUI is useful for couples when the concerns are low sperm count, altered sperm motility, thick or scant cervical mucus, or a generally hostile vaginal environment, or when a male donor is needed.
- IUI can be performed with or without ovulation-enhancing medications. HCG is prescribed to ensure ovulation within 34 to 40 hours.

Gamete Intrafallopian Transfer

- Gamete intrafallopian transfer (GIFT) is a three-step procedure that involves removing the eggs, combining them with sperm, and immediately placing them in the fallopian tubes, where the egg is fertilized.

- The woman is given follicle-stimulating drugs to increase her chances of producing multiple eggs. The eggs are collected via aspiration and mixed with sperm.
- Using laparoscopy, the combined egg and sperm mixture is placed in the fallopian tubes.
- GIFT is an option only if the woman has a healthy uterus and fallopian tubes.

In Vitro Fertilization

- In vitro fertilization (IVF) involves removing the eggs via aspiration, combining them with sperm in the laboratory, and creating a laboratory environment that enables fertilization and early development of the embryo. If fertilization occurs successfully, the embryo is transferred into the uterus. A 2-hour rest period following the procedure is recommended.
- Intracytoplasmic sperm injection (ICSI) involves obtaining the eggs via aspiration and inserting a single sperm through the zona pellucida (the external covering of the egg) or into the cytoplasm of the egg. ICSI is used with couples with male factor infertility problems, including poor motility, poor quality, inability to penetrate the egg or obstructive azoospermia caused by previous vasectomy, scarring from prior infections, or congenital absence of the vas deferens.
- Sperm for ICSI are retrieved through normal ejaculation, vasectomy reversal, or needle aspiration.
- Zygote intrafallopian transfer (ZIFT), also known as tubal embryo transfer (TET), is similar to IVF except that the fertilized egg is transferred into the fallopian tubes by laparoscopy. This is an option for couples who have failed prior efforts with ovarian stimulation and intrauterine insemination.
- Preimplantation genetic diagnosis (PGD) is a procedure whereby the embryos created in IVF are tested for genetic defects. The purpose is to allow the parents to make the decision about whether to continue with implantation or discard the embryos. This procedure usually is performed in cases in which the man or woman is a known carrier of a specific disease condition, the woman is over 35, or there is a history of repeated miscarriage.

Clinical Pearl

Success rates for most of the assisted reproductive techniques are available at the Centers for Disease Control and Prevention (CDC) Web site. http://www.cdc.gov/reproductivehealth/ART02/index.htm http://www.cdc.gov/MMWR/preview/mmwrhtml/ss5504a1.htm Last accessed January 18, 2007.

22

Menopause

WHAT IS IT?

Definition

Meno is the root word for menses, and *pausis* means cessation. Menopause is the permanent cessation of menstrual activity.

Concepts

The principal circulating hormone during menopause is estrone; before menopause it is estradiol. Estrone converts to estradiol and vice versa, with approximately 15% of estradiol converting to estrone and 5% of estrone to estradiol. Primary estrogen production shifts from the ovaries to the adrenal glands and peripheral tissues. The adrenal gland increases production of androstenedione, which is converted to estrone by aromatase enzyme, found in considerable quantities in fat cells. Aromatase also converts testosterone to estrone.

WHO GETS IT?

Every woman will go through menopause, which is a natural process of aging. The entire period covering the transition from perimenopause to menopause and beyond is called the *climacteric.*

Technical Note
Menopause can be achieved prematurely by hysterectomy, chemotherapy, radiation therapy, and premature ovarian failure.

ETIOLOGY

The number of ovarian follicles declines from approximately 6 million at birth to approximately 10,000 at menopause. The ovarian follicles are responsible for production of estrogen and progesterone. With the decline in the number of follicles, a corresponding decline in the levels of estrogen and progesterone occurs.

SIGNS AND SYMPTOMS

Some women transition through the menopause with minimal or no symptoms; for others, the symptoms are debilitating. Estrogen receptor sites have been found on the surface of virtually every tested cell, including the retina, the skin, and various organs and organ systems. This might explain the broad range of symptoms experienced by women during the transition. Primary menopausal symptoms include the following:

- Vasomotor (hot flashes, night sweats)
- Genitourinary (atrophy, bladder infections, prolapse [including feelings of fullness or a lump in the vagina], dragging sensation in the abdomen and lower back, changes in vaginal discharge, difficulty with coitus, and cystitis)
- Psychosocial/psychologic (depression, mood swings, sleep disturbances)
- Cardiovascular (arrhythmia, atherosclerosis)
- Skeletal (bone mineral density/osteoporosis)

Technical Note

Symptoms that have been associated with menopause but that may occur primarily as an aging effect include the following:
- Changes in appearance (weight gain, thinning hair, wrinkles)
- Changes in cognition (diminished concentration)

DIAGNOSIS

Amenorrhea for a period of 12 months signals menopause.

Definitive diagnosis is by blood analysis of follicle-stimulating hormone (FSH). As ovarian production of estrogen declines, the anterior pituitary produces more FSH in an attempt to increase estrogen production. Levels of FSH that exceed 40 mIU/ml are an indication of menopause. Confirmation via hormonal levels requires more than one FSH analysis.

Vasomotor (Hot Flashes/Flushes, Night Sweats)
MANAGEMENT

The cause of hot flashes remains unknown. Proposed causes include increased hypothalamic and pituitary activity in an effort to enhance FSH production and heat loss at the level of the arterioles instead of the capillaries and venules.

Lifestyle

- Keeping a diary of diet and lifestyle factors that occur with hot flashes might elicit a pattern.
- Dressing in layers.
- Exercising, such as walking and yoga.
- Identifying and avoiding hot flash triggers. Known triggers include stress, heat, caffeine, tomatoes, and berries.
- Taking supplements of the bioflavonoids naturally found in citrus fruit may help relieve hot flashes.
- Ensure adequate levels of fiber. Two to three servings of soy iso-flavones and other sources of fiber per day are recommended.
- Cruciferous vegetables (broccoli, cauliflower, cabbage, kale, and collard greens) are sources of indole-3-carbinol, which facilitates liver metabolism for the less potent 2-OH estrogen derivative.

Technical Note
Bioflavonoids have been identified as hot flash triggers in some women.

Vitamins, Minerals, and Herbs

- Black cohosh (RemiFemin), 500 to 1000 mg of the dry herb or 20 to 40 mg of the extract daily. There is evidence that black cohosh works better when combined with other herbs such as red clover (approximately 40 mg/day) and soy isoflavones (45 to 50 mg/day).
- Vitamin E (400 to 800 IU daily).

Acupressure

Acupressure points for hot flashes include triple warmer 3, bladder 66, stomach 43, and kidney 3.

Spinal Manipulation

- Low-force adjustments to ensure proper alignment. L1, L2 for ovarian innervation and C0/C1 and L5/S1 to ensure proper parasympathetic stimulation.

Bioidentical Hormones

These are hormones manufactured to have the same molecular structure as those naturally produced in the body. An individualized approach is taken in using the information from the hormonal assay to compound specific dosages of estrogen, testosterone, and DHEA. Careful monitoring via evaluation of symptoms and subsequent hormonal panels is required.

MEDICATIONS

- Estrogen or estrogen plus progesterone. Low-dose estrogen (i.e., doses less than or equal to 0.3 mg of conjugated equine estrogen, less than or equal to 0.5 mg of oral micronized estradiol, less than or equal to 25 mcg of transdermal estradiol, or less than or equal to 2.5 mcg of ethinyl estradiol) have been shown to be effective in most women. Some women require higher doses. Estrogen therapy at doses equivalent to 0.625 mg of conjugated equine estrogen increases the risk for stroke, deep venous thrombosis, and pulmonary embolism, and, when combined with progestin medroxyprogesterone acetate, results in increased risk for coronary events and breast cancer.
- Progesterone only. Megestrol acetate, formerly used for breast cancer treatment, helps to reduce hot flashes.
- Synthetic steroids such as tibolone.
- Antidepressants. Low doses of certain antidepressants may be helpful, including venlafaxine (Effexor XR) and selective serotonin reuptake inhibitors (SSRIs) such as paroxetine (Paxil), fluoxetine (Prozac), and citalopram (Celexa).

- Clonidine, a medication typically used for high blood pressure, has been shown to decrease hot flashes in breast cancer survivors.

Technical Note

Combined estrogen and testosterone use increases breast cancer risk.

Genitourinary Atrophy/Prolapse

Estrogen's functions include maintaining collagen levels in the skin and epithelial tissues, increasing vascular supply and fluid content of tissues, and enhancing tissue integrity.

Some of the changes resulting from menopausal decline of estrogen include the following:

- Atrophy of the vaginal, cervical, and uterine tissues
- Changes in the consistency and quantity of vaginal lubrication
- Thinning and drying out of the vulvar and vaginal tissues
- Prolapse
- Increased susceptibility to infection

MANAGEMENT

Technical Note

Uterine and urinary bladder prolapse of menopause is best managed prophylactically. Strategies include prenatal and postnatal exercises such as Kegel exercises, knee-chest pulls on the slant board, gluteal contractions, pelvic rock while squeezing a pillow between the knees, correcting for leg length discrepancies, appropriate management of birth to prevent excessive tearing of the perineum, and ensuring that the pelvis is in proper alignment. Predisposing factors such as obesity and a chronic cough should be controlled. Heavy lifting and repeated stair climbing should be avoided.

Lifestyle Management

- Avoid medications that cause mucosal dryness, including antihistamines and decongestants
- Kegel exercises (see Appendix)
- Increased sexual activity (increase foreplay)

Vitamins, Minerals, and Herbs

- Chaste berry 150 to 500 mg/day
- Black cohosh 500 to 1000 mg of the dry herb or 20 to 40 mg of the extract
- Zinc 15 mg/day and high-zinc foods such as seafood (especially oysters), red meat and poultry, wheat germ, oats and other whole grains, beans, nuts, and fortified cereals
- Manganese
- Vitamin C

Local Vaginal Therapies

- Flaxseed oil as a lubricant
- Vaginal estrogen creams such as Estrace
- Vaginal estrogen ring such as Estring
  These may be contraindicated in women with a history of estrogen-dependent conditions such as fibroids, breast cancer, and uterine cancer.

Spinal and Pelvic Manipulation

Assess for leg length deficiency, adjust to correct pelvic misalignment, leg length deficiency, and lumbar subluxations.

Massage

Balance the muscles of the pelvis.

Physical Therapy

- Pelvic floor (Kegel) exercises
- Electrical therapies to increase the tone of the pelvic floor

Other

- Devices, including the pessary
- Surgery may be recommended in severe cases

Atrophic Vaginitis

WHAT IS IT?

Atrophic vaginitis is inflammation of the vaginal epithelium, usually caused by a decrease in estrogen. It is a common manifestation of genitourinary atrophy.

WHO GETS IT?

Atrophic vaginitis occurs primarily in postmenopausal women, but it can occur in women who have had a hysterectomy, are breast-feeding, are on progesterone-only birth control medications, or have premature ovarian failure. It occurs rarely in premenarcheal children.

ETIOLOGY

Estrogens are responsible for keeping the vaginal tissue hydrated, collagen filled, and elastic. Diminished levels of estrogen, such as occurs in menopause, causes the vaginal tissue to become atrophic, thin, and easily traumatized.

SIGNS AND SYMPTOMS

- Vaginal burning
- Pruritus
- Bleeding or spotting
- Pinkish discharge
- Dyspareunia

DIAGNOSIS

- Pelvic examination, which reveals atrophic changes in the lower genital tract. The vaginal epithelium appears thin and transparent with decreased rugal folds. It also may appear reddened. The vaginal discharge may be thin, watery, and bloodstained.

- Microscopic evaluation of the vaginal discharge may reveal inflammatory cells and epithelial cells.
- It is atypical to find *Trichomonas vaginalis, Gardnerella vaginalis,* or other pathogenic agents.

Clinical Pearl

Some of the symptoms of atrophic vaginitis may occur with other, more serious conditions such as endometrial cancer and vaginal cancer. Women with these symptoms should be evaluated first for these conditions.

MANAGEMENT

Lifestyle

- Regular sexual activity, to improve blood circulation to the vagina.
- Topical application of flaxseed oil.
- Some authorities recommend topical application of cocoa butter, beeswax, or mineral oil to aid with sexual activity. These should be used with caution because they may clog the pores.
- Ingestion of foods high in phytoestrogens such as soy, parsley, linseed, fennel, and celery.
- Eicosapentaenoic acid/docosahexaenoic acid (EPA/DHA) and other fish oils added to the diet.

Medications

- Topical application of intravaginal estrogen cream.
- Estrogen replacement therapy.

Clinical Pearl

Estrogen therapy may be contraindicated in women with a history of liver disease, deep vein thrombosis, thrombophlebitis, or fibroids.

Psychosocial/Psychologic Aspects of Menopause

Menopause is a time of transition that for some is liberating, but for others is frightening and even depressing. Societal views on aging often affect this transition. In societies in which aging is viewed positively, menopausal symptoms do not appear to occur as frequently or with the same severity. It should be noted, however, that these frequently are societies in which individuals are generally more physically active, and the diet is rich in cruciferous vegetables, fiber, soy-based products, and lignans. The added benefits of these products in modulating the hormonal transition have been documented.

The psychologic and psychosocial changes in menopause are due in part to the changes in hormonal levels of estrogen and progesterone and to concentration of the neurotransmitters. Estrogens facilitate the release of the neurotransmitter norepinephrine in the brain and may decrease the action of monoamine oxidase. Estrogen also may aid in the functioning of serotonin, dopamine, and gamma-aminobutyric acid type A (GABAA), all of which have effects on the individual's mental state.

MANAGEMENT

- Lifestyle factors such as sleeping in the dark and avoiding the use of night-lights. This aids the function of the pineal gland, which is responsible for melatonin synthesis. Melatonin is needed for sleep.
- Diet. Ensure adequate intake of the omega-3 fatty acids, soy isoflavones, red clover, and lignans (e.g., flaxseed).
- Exercise—mild to moderate intensity several times a week.

Vitamins and Herbs

- Hormonal system modulators such as chaste berry 150 to 500 mg/day.
- S-adenosyl-L-methionine (SAMe) 800 mg/day in split doses to enhance serotonin function.
- St. John's wort is known to inhibit serotonin uptake in the brain and to inhibit the enzyme catechol-O-methyltransferase, which degrades the neurotransmitter dopamine. As with any herb, caution is necessary because St. John's wort may decrease the efficacy of medications such as the protease inhibitors used for human immunodeficiency virus (HIV), the theophyllines used for asthma, blood thinners such as Coumadin, and some chemotherapeutic agents. Patients who have

been taking St. John's wort should not discontinue the herb abruptly because this may increase systemic levels of other medications.
- Manage for adrenal fatigue, symptoms of which include depression, loss of libido, and total exhaustion.
  - Supplementation with dehydroepiandrosterone (DHEA) is advisable in some cases. DHEA converts to testosterone, which converts to estrogen, resulting in an increased estrogen load. This is of benefit to women whose symptoms are associated with estrogen insufficiency; however, the potential negative impact of the increased estrogen load on estrogen-related cancers should not be minimized. Dosage recommendations range from 10 to 100 mg/day. Levels should be monitored with blood analysis.
  - Licorice root as a tea or tincture also can be used to support adrenal function.
  - Ashwaganda root may also support adrenal function.

Technical Note
- Licorice root can increase blood pressure and cause water retention.
- The herbs fennel and sage also have been used to decrease hot flashes.

Medications

Antidepressants. The selective serotonin reuptake inhibitors (SSRIs) such as fluoxetine (Prozac), sertraline (Zoloft), and paroxetine (Paxil) frequently are used.

For More Information

- Bladder infections in menopause—see Chapter 20.
- Cardiovascular involvement—see Chapter 8.
- Osteoporosis—see Chapter 24.

23

Menorrhagia

WHAT IS IT?

Menorrhagia is excessive menstrual bleeding. It can be described as menses that lasts longer than 7 days; menses that occurs more frequently than every 21 days; menses that is heavy enough to require lifestyle modifications; excessive clotting; or intermenstrual bleeding.

WHO GETS IT?

Women of childbearing age, although it is more commonly seen in women in their thirties and forties.

ETIOLOGY

Common causes of menorrhagia include the following:
- Fibroids
- Endometriosis
- Abortion or threatened miscarriage
- Use of some intrauterine devices (IUDs) for birth control

Clinical Pearl
Progesterone-containing IUDs such as the Mirena IUD may decrease menstrual flow.

- Pelvic inflammatory disease (PID)
- Uterine polyps
- Congenital uterine anomalies
- Stress

- Insufficient nutrient intake
- Some birth control pills
- Abnormal hormonal fluctuations
- Increased prostaglandin activity
- Medications such as the anticoagulants and some anti-inflammatory agents may contribute to prolonged or heavy menstrual bleeding

SIGNS AND SYMPTOMS

- Excessive menstrual bleeding that may or may not be accompanied by pain

DIAGNOSIS

- Careful, comprehensive history
- Assessment for iron deficiency anemia
- Assessment for reproductive tract cancers
- Pelvic examination and Papanicolaou (Pap) smear
- Complete blood count (CBC)
- Endometrial biopsy
- Dilation and curettage (D&C) if the biopsy is normal and bleeding persists
- Ultrasound to evaluate for fibroids and ovarian cysts/tumors
- Hysterosalpingogram (HSG)
- Hysteroscopy

MANAGEMENT

Identify and manage the causative factor:
- Lifestyle
- Diet
  - Foods high in beta-carotene, including watermelon and other brightly colored fruits and vegetables such as sweet potatoes, red yams, peppers, carrots, beets, and squash
  - Foods high in iron, including fish, poultry, red meats, green leafy vegetables, and legumes

Spinal Manipulation

Spinal manipulation at the thoracolumbar junction and sacrum. Anecdotal evidence has reported shorter bleeding times with adjustment at S2 following cervical cauterization.

Medications

Medications currently used for menorrhagia include the following:

- Birth control pills help regulate the timing and intensity of each cycle. Either the combined pill or the progesterone-only pills may be used. These help maintain a uterine lining that is less vascular, resulting in lighter periods.
- Depo-Provera, the progestin-only birth control injection administered every 3 months, reduces the thickness of the endometrial lining, thereby reducing blood loss.
- Gonadotropin-releasing hormone (GnRH) agonists such as Lupron and Nafarelin create a menopausal state by depleting follicle-stimulating hormone (FSH) and luteinizing hormone (LH) secretion from the pituitary, thereby reducing or eliminating menstrual flow. GnRH agonists are more commonly used to minimize blood loss during myomectomy and rarely are used as a long-term strategy for menorrhagia management.
- The nonsteroidal antiinflammatory drugs (NSAIDs) and the prostaglandin synthetase inhibitors such as Naprosyn, Ibuprofen, Advil, and Motrin reduce bleeding and modulate the pain sometimes associated with menorrhagia.
- Antibiotics are administered to treat menorrhagia caused by PID.

PROCEDURES

- Endometrial ablation to destroy the entire internal lining of the uterus
- Endometrial resection to remove the lining of the uterus
- Insertion of progestin-releasing IUDs, which release small amounts of levonergesterel locally into the uterus, thereby reducing menstrual blood loss
- Laparoscopy or myomectomy if fibroids or endometriosis are identified as the causative factor
- Hysterectomy or hysterectomy with bilateral salpingo-oophorectomy

---

Clinical Pearl

The most common complication of menorrhagia is iron deficiency anemia. Iron is needed by the blood to make hemoglobin, the oxygen-carrying component of red blood cells. Menorrhagia is the most common cause of anemia in premenopausal women.

Symptoms of iron deficiency anemia include weakness, fatigue, shortness of breath, brittle nails, tinnitus, headaches, rapid heart rate, light-headedness, memory loss, general mental confusion, irritability, pale skin, and restless legs syndrome.

Management of iron deficiency anemia may require the following:

- Dietary alterations (foods high in iron, including liver and other red meats, green leafy vegetables, fish, beans, fortified cereals and breads, chicken, and turkey)
- Iron supplementation (up to 45 mg daily)
- Vitamin C to enhance iron absorption
- The herb yellow dock is a good source of iron

Clinical Pearl

Menorrhagia in a postmenopausal woman who is not on combined hormonal replacement therapy is always a cause for concern because of the risk for vaginal or uterine cancer.

24

Osteoporosis

WHAT IS IT?

- Osteoporosis is a decline in the mass of bone (*osteo*–bone, *porous*–passage, *osis*–condition).
- Osteoblasts make bone.
- Osteoclasts resorb (dissolve) bone.
- A primary function of estrogen is to inhibit osteoclastic activity. During menopause, estrogen levels decline, osteoclast-mediated bone resorption is uninhibited, and osteoblastic function declines, resulting in osteoporosis.

WHO GETS IT?

Osteoporosis is influenced by the following factors:
- Hereditary factors/genetics. Asian women, and Caucasian women with a slight frame, are at higher risk.
- Lack of or inadequate weight-bearing exercise.
- Dietary factors, including inadequate calcium intake and excessive phosphate intake. Phosphates found in many soda drinks compete with calcium and can force the expulsion of calcium.
- Inadequate exposure to sunlight, which can impede vitamin D synthesis. Vitamin D is necessary for calcium absorption.

Clinical Pearl

Deficiencies in vitamin D can be compounded by living in a Nordic climate, being dark skinned, and wearing clothing that covers the entire body.

- Prolonged use of medications such as blood thinners, thyroid hormone, glucocorticoids, antiseizure medications, and gonadotropin-releasing hormone (GnRH) agonists such as Lupron can induce osteoporosis.
- Aluminum-containing antacids such as Maalox and Mylanta may increase the risk for osteoporosis.
- Early-onset menopause as a result of a hysterectomy or an oophorectomy.
- Illnesses such as Celiac disease and Crohn's disease interfere with gastric absorption of calcium and other minerals and predispose to osteoporosis.
- Hormonal imbalances brought on by conditions such as hyperthyroidism, Cushing's syndrome, female athlete triad, and hyperparathyroidism predispose to osteoporosis.

SIGNS AND SYMPTOMS

- Spinal pain as a result of compression fractures and microfractures
- Hip pain
- Loss of height
- Stooped posture
- Dowager's hump

DIAGNOSIS

Screening Procedures

- Bone mineral density (BMD) screening/assessment is a relatively noninvasive procedure that also can be used to monitor treatment efficacy. BMD measurement is given as a T-score and a Z-score. The T-score is the deviation from the mean bone density of healthy young adults of the same gender and ethnicity, and the Z-score is the deviation from the mean bone density of adults of the same age and gender.
- Dual-energy x-ray absorptiometry (DEXA) scans the entire body and measures BMD. From the results, physicians assess the risk for fracture in the hip, spine, and wrist. Radiation exposure is low and time commitment minimal (approximately 5 minutes). DEXA can be used to monitor changes in bone density during treatment.

- Quantitative computed tomography (QCT) measures bone density in the hip and spine and produces a three-dimensional image that shows true volume density. The radiation level in QCT is 10 times higher than in DEXA.
- Peripheral bone density testing uses ultrasound to identify bone loss in a localized area such as the heel or hand.
- X-ray. Unfortunately, osteoporosis does not show up on regular spinal x-rays until there is a 30% loss of bone.

MANAGEMENT

Lifestyle Management

Recognizing and managing the factors that contribute to osteoporosis will help to prevent it or modulate its severity. These include the following:
- Get adequate exposure to sunlight.
- Consume adequate amounts of calcium in the diet.
- Avoid excessive intake of calcium-excreting products such as phosphates in some sodas.
- Because bones mineralize fully only when placed under stress, initiate weight-bearing exercise at an early age.

Diet

Include additional calcium along with magnesium in the diet.

Clinical Pearl

Most adults lose the ability to make the enzyme lactase by age 45 (and much younger in some ethnic populations). Most black people lose the ability to make lactase by age 18; therefore milk is not an ideal source of calcium in black adults. Yogurt and buttermilk are suitable sources of calcium for adults because they are fermented products, made with cultures that break down the lactose. Cheese is a protein curd that does not contain lactose and also is appropriate.

- Consume a diet rich in fruits and vegetables, especially green vegetables.
- Whole grains, such as brown rice, millet, buckwheat, whole wheat, triticale, quinoa, rye, legumes, and leafy vegetables,

Type of calcium supplement	Easily absorbed	Calcium content (%)	Other benefits	Disadvantages
Calcium Ascorbate	Yes	10%	Vitamin C is the other component	
Calcium Aspartate	Yes	20%		
Calcium Carbonate	Not always Should be taken with food for maximum absorption.	40%	Inexpensive source of calcium. Has antacid effect.	Has antacid effect. Can interfere with digestion. May not be well absorbed in people with insufficient output of stomach acid. Can cause gas.
Calcium Citrate	Yes	2%	Can be absorbed by those with poor digestion. Reduces risk for kidney stones.	Larger molecule is bulkier than calcium carbonate, thus requiring more tablets/capsules to achieve the same dosage as calcium carbonate.
Calcium Lactate	Yes	15%	May contain milk and/or yeast byproducts.	May contain milk and or yeast byproducts. Larger molecule is bulkier than calcium carbonate, thus requiring more tablets/capsules to achieve the same dosage as calcium carbonate.
Calcium amino acid chelate	Yes	10%–20%	Lactose intolerance	May be incorrectly made as a soy blend.

Bone Meal	Yes	39%	Contains many of the minerals needed for bone.	May contain lead, arsenic, cadmium, and other unidentified minerals. Some of the organic constituents are destroyed by heat during processing. More expensive.
Microcrystalline Hydroxyapatite Concentrate (MCHC)	Yes/No	25%	Contains collagen and several of the other minerals needed for healthy bone formation, including phosphorous, fluoride, mg, Fe, Zn, cu, ma.	
Calcium phosphate Coral calcium, oyster shell, calcium dolomite, and bone meal	No	38%	Is essentially calcium carbonate. Better to use purified calcium carbonate products (see above).	Least likely to cause constipation. Blocks absorption of iron and other minerals. May contain high levels of lead and other impurities.

are rich in calcium. Whole grains and legumes also are rich in magnesium, which helps bone to incorporate calcium.

- Minimize high-protein diets because they can cause larger than normal calcium excretion, thereby increasing the potential for bone loss.

Vitamins, Minerals, and Herbs

- Calcium 1000 to 1500 mg/day
- Vitamin D (minimum of 400 IU/day)
- Herbs for bone health, including oat straw and horsetail

Acupressure

Acupressure points for bone health include kidney 1 between the second and third metatarsals, kidney 3 on the medial side of the foot behind the tibia, and bladder 64 on the little toe.

Spinal Manipulation

Low-force techniques should be used.

Physical Therapy

- Fall risk assessment and prevention
- Balance training
- Postural reeducation
- Spinal extensor strengthening
- Core muscle strengthening
- Pelvic floor training
- Weight-bearing exercises
- Hip flexor, erector spinae, and abdominal muscle stretching
- Pain management in the presence of fractures
  - Hydrotherapy when the patient has pain from recent vertebral fracture or postural and balance problems
  - Transcutaneous electrical nerve stimulation (TENS)
  - Interferential therapy
  - Heat therapies
  - Acupuncture
  - Aromatherapy
  - Reflex therapy

- Relaxation techniques
- Bracing

MEDICATIONS

The 2006 position statement of the North American Menopause Society provides the following guidelines for medication management of osteoporosis in postmenopausal women:

- Bisphosphonates are the first-line drugs for treating postmenopausal women with osteoporosis. Alendronate and risedronate reduce the risk of both vertebral and nonvertebral fractures.
- The selective estrogen-receptor modulator (SERM) raloxifene is most often considered in postmenopausal women with low bone mass or younger postmenopausal women with osteoporosis who are at greater risk of spine fracture than hip fracture. It prevents bone loss and reduces the risk of vertebral fractures.
- Teriparatide (parathyroid hormone [PTH] 1–34) is reserved for treating women at high risk of fracture, including those with very low BMD (T-score worse than 3.0) or with a previous vertebral fracture. PTH improves BMD and reduces the risk of new vertebral and nonvertebral fractures.
- Calcitonin is not a first-line drug for postmenopausal osteoporosis treatment, because its fracture efficacy is not strong and its BMD effects are less than those of other agents. However, it is an option for women with osteoporosis who are more than 5 years beyond menopause.

25

Pelvic Inflammatory Disease

WHAT IS IT?

Pelvic inflammatory disease (PID), as described by the Centers for Disease Control, is a general term that refers to infection of the uterus, fallopian tubes, and other reproductive organs. It is a common and serious complication of some sexually transmitted diseases (STDs), especially chlamydia and gonorrhea. PID can damage the fallopian tubes and tissues in and near the uterus and ovaries. Untreated PID can lead to serious consequences, including infertility, ectopic pregnancy, abscess formation, and chronic pelvic pain.

WHO GETS IT?

PID affects as many as 1 million women every year in the United States. It occurs primarily during the menstruating years, most commonly in women under 25 years of age.

ETIOLOGY

- Organisms migrate from the vagina and cervix into the uterus and pelvis. Infection spreads along the mucosal surface of the endometrium to the fallopian tubes, onto the ovaries, and into the peritoneum.
- About 10% of PID is iatrogenically induced as a result of an abortion, intrauterine device (IUD) insertion, or dilation and curettage (D&C).
- PID also can result from transperitoneal spread of infection from a ruptured appendix or intraabdominal abscess.

- The two most common pathogens implicated in PID are *Neisseria gonorrhoeae* and *Chlamydia trachomatis*.
- Risk factors for PID include the following:
  - Age less than 25
  - Sexual activity (one in eight sexually active adolescent girls will develop acute PID)
  - Menstruation
  - Prior history of PID
  - Use of the IUD as a contraceptive device
  - Recent instrumentation or genital tract invasive procedures
  - Douching
  - Procedures or processes that involve dilation of the cervical canal, including menses, childbirth, abortion, miscarriage, D&C, and IUD insertion

SIGNS AND SYMPTOMS

Acute Pelvic Inflammatory Disease

- Symptoms begin during or immediately after menstruation
- Presenting complaint often is dull lower abdominal pain less than 7 days in duration and exacerbated by movement or sexual intercourse
- Increased vaginal discharge
- Fever or chills
- Nausea and vomiting
- Right upper quadrant abdominal pain referring to the corresponding shoulder and perihepatitis with mild liver function test abnormalities (Fitz-Hugh–Curtis syndrome)
- Rebound tenderness
- Fatigue or generalized weakness
- Dyspareunia
- Urinary frequency and urgency

Subacute Pelvic Inflammatory Disease

- Low back pain
- Symptoms as in acute PID, but mild to moderate severity and slower onset
- Symptoms may persist for some time before the patient seeks treatment

Chronic Pelvic Inflammatory Disease

- Constant or intermittent low back pain
- Constant or intermittent abdominal pain
- Persistent low-grade infection
- History of acute infection that never completely resolved
- Menstrual irregularities
- Infection of Bartholin's glands

DIAGNOSIS

- By signs and symptoms
- By differential diagnosis
- Ectopic pregnancy—pregnancy test, abdominal ultrasound, and serum human chorionic gonadotropin (HCG) that does not double in 48 hours
- Appendicitis—rebound tenderness, fever, nausea and vomiting, leukocytosis, fever; location, onset, and intensity of pain
- Timing—symptoms often begin during or immediately after menstruation
- Pelvic examination that reveals pain with movement of the cervix, colored pus discharge from the cervix, and pain or a mass in the adnexa
- Leukocytosis and erythrocyte sedimentation rate (ESR)
- History of IUD insertion or abortion
- STD screening that reveals yellow or green discharge

Technical Note
Women in high-risk categories (i.e., sexually active young girls and girls and women with multiple partners) should be routinely screened.

MANAGEMENT

- Broad-spectrum antibiotics
- Hospitalization if symptoms do not improve within 48 to 72 hours with oral antibiotics
- Pelvic rest (i.e., bed rest and sexual abstinence)
- Fluids
- The partner should be treated for STDs
- Surgery may be warranted

Technical Note

The risk of PID leading to scarring in the fallopian tubes and subsequent infertility necessitates an aggressive approach to the management of PID. It is this author's opinion that PID should be managed primarily with antibiotics.

Adjunctive treatments for chronic PID might include the following:

- Garlic. The clove is peeled and crushed, wrapped in gauze, lubricated with K-Y jelly or garlic oil, and inserted into the vagina for several hours or overnight.
- Ginger root poultices applied topically to decrease pain, dissolve adhesions, and eliminate toxins.
- Castor oil compresses placed over the abdomen.
- Raspberry leaf tea, which aids in improving or maintaining healthy functioning of the reproductive organs.
- Low-force adjustive techniques such as activator and Logan basic.
- Multivitamins and minerals that support the immune system.

PREVENTION

- Extra care should be taken whenever the cervix is dilated. Nothing should be placed into the vaginal vault for 3 weeks after miscarriage, abortion, or D&C; for 6 weeks after childbirth; and during menses.
- Wipe from front to back after bowel movements.
- Seek prompt treatment of all vaginal infections.
- Practice "safer sex" techniques.
- Abstain from sexual activity.

26

Perimenopause

WHAT IS IT?

Perimenopause is the phase prior to menopause. For many women this can begin as early as age 35.

At its best, a woman may not notice that she is transitioning into menopause, because her life is in balance and the transition occurs gradually. At its worst, perimenopause may be a time of moderate to severe adolescence-like symptoms because the adrenal glands, ovaries, and pituitary gland all are transitioning.

WHO GETS IT?

Women experience perimenopausal symptoms in their thirties and forties.

ETIOLOGY

- Perimenopause is a normal phase of transition. It is marked by some of the same symptoms that occur during the other time of major hormonal transition (i.e., adolescence). The hormonal environment in perimenopause is tumultuous, unlike menopause, which is serene and steady.
- Perimenopausal symptoms may be compounded by factors such as adrenal fatigue, anovulatory cycles, and poor dietary habits.

Adrenal Fatigue

- The demands of work, family, children, aging parents, and society at large place undue stresses on many women. The result is a perpetual fight/fright cycle. The adrenal gland, which was designed to function only in times of danger, functions constantly, releasing norepinephrine and epinephrine from the adrenal medulla and corticosteroids, mineralocorticoids, and androgens from the adrenal cortex.

- The mineralocorticoids (primarily aldosterone) regulate the balance of minerals (sodium, potassium, and magnesium) in the cells. Stress triggers the release of aldosterone, which raises blood pressure by its action on cells to hold onto sodium and lose potassium. Long-term release of stress levels of mineralocorticoids can cause a potassium deficiency and a magnesium imbalance, as well as chronic water retention and high blood pressure. The resultant magnesium insufficiency as noted by red blood cell magnesium levels can affect many of the enzyme-driven metabolic pathways in the body.

- In addition, the adrenal cortex makes all the sex hormones in small amounts and dehydroepiandrosterone (DHEA) in large amounts. DHEA is important to the growth and repair of protein tissues and is a precursor to androstenediol, testosterone, and the estrogens. It is not a precursor to progesterone, aldosterone, pregnenolone, or the cortisols. Alterations to the normal production of the hormones of the adrenal cortex can predispose to multiple symptoms of perimenopause, including aggression and anger from too much testosterone, passivity, oversensitivity, mental confusion and agitation from too much estrogen, and depression from too little estrogen or progesterone.

Anovulatory Cycles

Ovulation becomes increasingly infrequent, the follicular phase is extended, and estrogen levels remain sustained for longer periods. In the absence of ovulation, progesterone is not released in adequate quantities, and progesterone deficiency or estrogen dominance, or both, may result.

Poor Dietary Habits

- Inadequate intake or absorption of many vitamins and minerals (e.g., vitamins C, E, and A; beta-carotene; and iron) impairs the functioning of many organ systems.

- The result of these dietary, hormonal, and lifestyle aberrations is fatigue, high blood pressure, uterine fibroids, mood swings, and several other identified symptoms of the perimenopause.

SIGNS AND SYMPTOMS

- Increasing vaginal dryness
- Decreased libido
- Acne
- Generalized fatigue
- Increasing blood pressure
- Endometriosis
- Uterine fibroids
- Symptoms of increased cortisol, which include papery (thin) skin, weight gain around the midsection, memory loss, blood sugar imbalances, and muscle wasting
- Mood swings
- Chronic fatigue
- Diabetes
- Menorrhagia and other menstrual irregularities
- Hot flashes
- Sleep disturbances
- Bladder problems
- Loss of bone mineral density

DIAGNOSIS

Diagnosis of perimenopause is primarily by signs and symptoms. Blood hormonal assays and salivary tests can be performed to guide symptomatic management. There are no known tests to determine how long a woman will be in perimenopause.

MANAGEMENT

Lifestyle

- Exercise—a low- to medium-intensity exercise program
- Coping mechanisms such as biofeedback, yoga, and meditation
- Dietary management, including legumes, phytoestrogens, and filtered water; avoiding sources of xenoestrogens
- Management for insulin resistance

- A good multivitamin with adequate dosages of calcium, magnesium, and the essential fatty acids
- Soy isoflavones
- Psychosocial and psychologic factors such as decreasing stress, developing and nurturing support systems, and recognizing that perimenopause is a phase of transition that can be managed
- Short-term use of low-dose progesterone creams

Technical Note

Prolonged use of high-dose progesterone creams is not recommended. The potential risk of increasing the hormonal load, facilitating an estrogen-dominant state and predisposing to estrogen-sensitive conditions such as breast cancer, endometriosis, and fibroids, warrants caution.

Bioidentical Hormones

These are hormones manufactured to have the same molecular structure as those naturally produced in the body. An individualized approach is taken in using the information from the hormonal assay to compound specific dosages of estrogen, testosterone, and DHEA. Patients are monitored carefully via symptom evaluation and subsequent hormonal panels.

MEDICATIONS

Symptom-specific medications include antidepressants, blood sugar modulators, and hormones.

27

Polycystic Ovary Syndrome

WHAT IS IT?

Polycystic ovary syndrome (PCOS) is an umbrella term used to label a group of symptoms that all appear to be connected to the menstrual cycle and to have a strong correlation with insulin sensitivity. PCOS currently is the most common hormonal disorder among women of reproductive age in the United States, affecting 5% to 10% of women. Symptoms associated with PCOS include hirsutism, obesity, menstrual irregularities, infertility, and acne.

WHO GETS IT?

PCOS occurs primarily in the menstruating female. It commonly is diagnosed in women in their twenties but frequently begins during adolescence.

ETIOLOGY

Insulin Resistance

Failure of the cells to respond adequately to stimulus from insulin initiates a vicious cycle in which blood sugar levels rise and, in response, the pancreas accelerates insulin production. The increased insulin levels ultimately result in an en masse entry of blood sugars into the cells, a corresponding rapid drop in blood sugar levels, and a hypoglycemic state. The cycle repeats; the pancreas eventually becomes overextended and no longer is able to produce sufficient amounts of insulin, and diabetes results. Insulin resistance is marked by simultaneously elevated levels of blood sugars and blood insulin. Ingesting simple carbohydrates and high glycemic index foods can compound the problem because they cause a rapid rise in blood sugars.

Glucose from sugars is converted to energy in the cells; in the absence of this critical source of energy, fatigue and food cravings result.

The liver responds to the elevated blood sugar levels by rapidly converting the excess sugars to fat.

The excess fat results in increased hormone load as more estrogen is stored in fatty tissue and synthesized via the aromatase enzyme.

Aromatase enzyme synthesizes estrogen via the androstenedione pathway, which ultimately may result in excess testosterone.

Excess testosterone levels cause male distribution hair growth (on the chest and chin) and acne.

Ovarian Failure

The ovarian follicles mature but do not release an egg, resulting in cyst formation on and around the ovaries, which subsequently can cause infertility and amenorrhea.

SIGNS AND SYMPTOMS

- Amenorrhea or oligomenorrhea
- Obesity
- Infertility
- Acne
- Hirsutism
- Polycystic ovaries
- Pelvic pain
- Thinning hair
- Hair loss
- Insulin resistance
- Type 2 diabetes
- Elevated cholesterol and other lipid abnormalities
- Elevated blood pressure
- Cardiovascular disease

DIAGNOSIS

- A careful gynecologic history
- Vaginal or abdominal ultrasound of the ovaries to evaluate for multiple cysts (Figure 27-1)
- Blood chemistries, which may reveal the following:
  - Elevated levels of luteinizing hormone (LH)
  - Low-normal levels of follicle-stimulating hormone (FSH)
  - Elevated blood glucose
  - Hyperandrogenism
  - Elevated blood lipids
- Monitoring of the ovary's response to either a stimulatory dose of a gonadotropin-releasing hormone agonist such as leuprolide or a suppressive dose of medications such as dexamethasone

MANAGEMENT

Lifestyle

Diet

- Diet for insulin resistance: increased complex carbohydrates, high fiber intake, and low glycemic index foods such as mung beans, soybeans and other legumes, nuts, artichokes, garlic, onions, mangoes, whole grain breads and cereals, barley, brown rice, whole wheat pasta

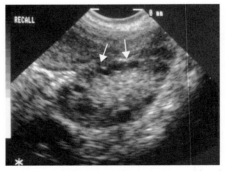

FIGURE 27-1 Transvaginal ultrasonography in a woman with polycystic ovary disease. The multiple subcapsular cysts, with their "string of pearls" appearance *(arrows),* are common in this syndrome. (From Hacker NF, Moore JG, Gambone JC: *Essentials of obstetrics and gynecology,* ed 4, Philadelphia, 2004, WB Saunders.)

- Avoid/decrease simple carbohydrates, including sodas, cookies, and candy
- Avoid trans fats
- Avoid food allergens

Exercise. Mild to moderate exercise is recommended. Intense exercise training may increase the symptoms of PCOS.

Miscellaneous. Applying progesterone creams to the inner wrist and upper chest during the luteal phase is intended to induce menstrual bleeding.

Spinal Manipulation

Spinal manipulation, particularly to the segments that innervate the ovaries.

Massage Therapies

Muscle stripping techniques to the adductor muscles may help to restore monthly bleeding.

Nutritional Supplementation

- EPA/DHA in dosages of 400 to 1000 mg daily
- For oligomenorrhea, chaste berry extract 20 mg one to three times daily

Medications

Treatments for PCOS typically are based on symptoms, taking into consideration whether the patient wants to conceive or needs contraception.

- Metformin, used primarily in diabetes, also is being used to manage insulin resistance
- Birth control pills to produce monthly bleeding, to protect against endometrial cancer, and to decrease testosterone concentrations
- Fertility medications
- Antiandrogenic medications

28

Pregnancy

WHAT IS IT?

Pregnancy is the development and maturation of a fertilized egg. The fertilized egg migrates through the fallopian tube to the uterine cavity and implants in the endometrium. The process from fertilization in the tubes to implantation in the uterine cavity is approximately 6 days. Following implantation, and over a period of several weeks, the lining of the uterus will change morphologically to become the decidua, which further differentiates to become the placenta. The placenta provides nourishment for the developing embryo for approximately 9 months.

SIGNS AND SYMPTOMS

First Trimester

Maternal symptoms may include but are not limited to fatigue, increased urination, nausea and vomiting, generalized malaise, breast tenderness and enlargement, amenorrhea or oligomenorrhea, and increased abdominal girth.

Second Trimester

Maternal signs and symptoms may include but are not limited to noticeable increase in weight, greater fatigue, fluid retention, indigestion, food cravings, light-headedness, dizziness, heartburn, gas, constipation, varicose veins, hemorrhoids, and stretch marks. False labor pains (Braxton Hicks contractions) may begin to occur.

Third Trimester

Maternal signs and symptoms may include but are not limited to Braxton Hicks contractions, stretching in the lower ribs, painful rib subluxations, indigestion (as the abdominal cavity becomes increasingly cramped), difficulties sleeping, difficulties breathing, frequent urination, low back pain, medial thigh pain, symphysis pubis pain, groin pain, thigh pain, constipation, tingling and numbness in the hands and extremities, swelling in the feet, and anxiety.

Lightening is the slight descent of the uterus when the head of the fetus drops into the birth canal in preparation for delivery.

DIAGNOSIS

- The presence of human chorionic gonadotropin (HCG) in maternal serum or urine is indication of pregnancy. Beta HCG is detected in maternal serum and urine 8 to 10 days after conception when implantation has occurred and vascular connections have been established between the syncytiotrophoblast and the decidua. HCG is detectable in 98% of patients by day 11.
- By presenting signs and symptoms (see first trimester symptoms, p. 180).

Technical Note

HCG is a glycoprotein that is similar in structure to follicle-stimulating hormone and luteinizing hormone. The free beta subunit of HCG is degraded by enzymes in the kidney to a beta subunit core fragment, which is primarily detected in urine samples.

MANAGEMENT

This section briefly summarizes etiology and protocols for managing select conditions of pregnancy (Figure 28-1).

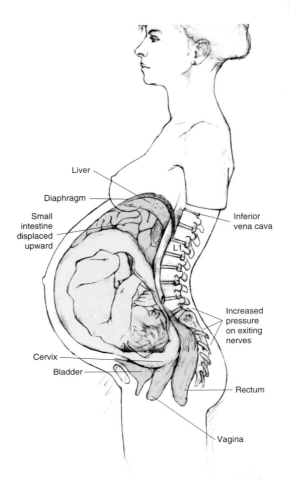

Liver

Diaphragm

Small
intestine
displaced
upward

Inferior
vena cava

L1

Increased
pressure
on exiting
nerves

Cervix

Bladder

Rectum

Vagina

FIGURE 28-1 This illustration shows the impressive degree to which the pregnant uterus displaces other abdominopelvic structures and puts pressure on important regions such as the pelvic diaphragm and the respiratory diaphragm. Venous return from pelvic and lower limb structures is made more difficult by pressure on the inferior vena cava, and women commonly develop hemorrhoids and varicose veins in the lower limbs. Breathing may be difficult because of pressure on the diaphragm and the inability to depress it fully to permit filling of the lungs. Back and lower limb pain is common because of pressure on exiting nerves of the lumbar and sacral plexuses. (From Mathers LH et al: *Clinical anatomy principles,* St Louis, 1996, Mosby.)

Bleeding Gums

Etiology
- Inadequate nutrition
- Poor dental hygiene

Management
- A good prenatal vitamin
- Vitamin C
- Meticulous dental hygiene
- Dental consultation if warranted

Breathing Difficulties

Etiology. The enlarging uterus restricts diaphragm excursion and predisposes toward anterior rotation of the pectoral girdle.

Management
- Trigger point therapy and deep tissue massage to the pectoralis major and minor, anterior, middle and posterior scalenes, levator scapula, sternocleido mastoid (SCM), rhomboids, serratus anterior, and trapezius muscles.
- Instructions to the patient in more lateral and posterior rib cage expansion techniques to foster deeper diaphragmatic breathing patterns.
- Diaphragm release techniques may be helpful.

Dehydration

Management. Dehydration in pregnancy is best managed prophylactically. The patient should be reminded regularly to monitor fluid intake and to drink a lot of water.

Diabetes (Gestational Diabetes)

Gestational diabetes—the more common form of diabetes in pregnancy—occurs in approximately 4% of pregnant women and is more common in women who are overweight, are over 35, or have a history of larger babies.

Etiology. The cause of gestational diabetes is unknown; however, it is thought that the placental hormones may block the action of the mother's insulin, first creating insulin resistance, and ultimately diabetes.

Risk factors
- Woman over 35 years old
- A previous baby weighing more than 9 lb
- Obesity
- African ancestry
- Hispanic ancestry
- Gestational diabetes in a previous pregnancy
- Recurrent infections

Diagnosis
- Glucose tolerance test
- One-hour postprandial glucose measurements
- Rate of weight gain

Management. Intense monitoring of nutritional practices, including the following:
- Carbohydrate content
- Caloric intake
- Fat content
- Ketone testing for patients on hypocaloric or carbohydrate-restricted diets
- Regular mild to moderate exercise
- Insulin or other medications

Clinical Pearl

Diagnosis of gestational diabetes frequently occurs during the second or third trimester, when the rate of weight gain typically is 3/4 to 1 lb per week. Many women are gaining almost 2 lb per week when they are diagnosed. Placing less emphasis on the total weight gain and greater emphasis on the rate of weight gain (i.e., to approximately 1 lb/wk) is an effective strategy.

Diastasis Recti Abdominis

Diastasis recti abdominis is separation of the fascial connection between the bellies of the right and left rectus abdominis muscles.

Etiology
- Unknown
- Familial
- Weakened core abdominal muscles

Symptoms
- None
- Bulging in the midline of the abdomen
- Separation at the midline of the abdomen
- Low back pain

Diagnosis
- Physical examination
- A separation of 1 inch or greater is observed in the "sit-up" position
- A visible bulge is observed

Management
- Core strengthening exercises
- Assisted abdominal crunches and abdominal exercises on the slant board
- Abdominal surgery if severe

Dizziness or Light-Headedness

Etiology. Dizziness or light-headedness can occur because of low blood pressure as a result of the decreased blood volume secondary to the rapid dilation of the blood vessels during the first half of the pregnancy. This is more common in the second trimester of pregnancy when the blood vessels have dilated in response to the hormones of pregnancy, but the blood volume is not yet enough to fill the blood vessels.

Management
- Take prenatal multivitamins
- Keep hydrated
- Avoid prolonged standing
- Rise slowly from the supine and seated positions
- Avoid long, hot showers; saunas; and hot tubs
- Eat foods rich in iron such as beans, spinach, red meats, and chicken

Fluid Retention Symptoms

Etiology
- Carpal tunnel syndrome if edema compromises the carpal tunnel
- Tarsal tunnel syndrome if edema results in compression of the tibial nerve in the tarsal tunnel
- Swollen feet and ankles

Technical Note
Rapid fluid retention may be an indication of preeclampsia in pregnancy.

Management

- Ensure adequate protein intake because inadequate protein intake is a cause of fluid retention.
- For carpal and tarsal tunnel symptoms, spinal manipulation is commonly needed along with physical therapy consisting of rehabilitative exercise, ultrasound and interferential therapies to the carpal and tarsal tunnels, trigger point therapy to the supporting muscles, and neutral wrist splints.
- Swollen feet and ankles may necessitate craniosacral release techniques to the pelvic diaphragm if the pelvic fascia is restricted.

Groin Pain

Etiology
- Misalignment of the symphysis pubis bone
- Symphysis pubis diastasis, which produces sharp and sometimes incapacitating pain
- Round ligament pain as the uterus enlarges during pregnancy

Management
- Realignment of the pubic ramus
- Massage and trigger point therapy to the pelvic muscles and round ligament
- Manipulation of the pelvis

Headaches

Etiology. Headaches in pregnancy can be caused by a myriad of factors, including the following:
- Hormonal effects on blood dilation
- Suboccipital muscle strain
- Strain and trigger points in the posterior cervical and upper back muscles
- Subluxation of the cervical and cervicothoracic vertebrae
- Elevated blood pressure or preeclampsia
- Overall stress and strain

Management
- Carefully identify and manage the contributing cause or causes
- Teach coping strategies

Heartburn

Etiology. Heartburn is the backward flow of stomach acids into the esophagus as a result of factors such as restrictions in the respiratory diaphragm, sluggish digestion, poor dietary choices, and an enlarging uterus.

Management
- Lifestyle
- Smaller meals eaten several times during the day
- Avoidance of known heartburn triggers
- Not lying down within 30 minutes of eating a meal
- Craniosacral therapy release techniques to the respiratory diaphragm
- Use of the hiatal hernia maneuver

Increased Vaginal Discharge

Etiology. Increased vaginal discharge is an almost universal occurrence during pregnancy and is due to turnover of the cells lining the vaginal vault. The hormonally induced thickening of the vaginal vault can cause leukorrhea, a thin, white, odorless discharge that is normal but still should be reported to the health care provider.

Management. This condition does not usually require treatment.

In Utero Constraint

In utero constraint is the term used to describe some of the external forces that obstruct the normal movements of the fetus. This constraint may prevent the developing fetus from achieving the head-down vertex position in preparation for vaginal birth. Breech presentation is a primary reason for many cesarean sections.

Etiology. The causes of in utero constraint are multiple and include sacrum subluxation, hypertonic muscles, stress, or fatigue in the mother.

Management. The Webster technique is used specifically for pregnant mothers in the third trimester to relieve the musculoskeletal causes of in utero constraint. It involves adjusting the sacrum for misalignment and gently massaging the round ligament (see Appendix for detailed description).

Low Back Pain

Almost half of all pregnant women experience some back pain, especially during the fifth through ninth months. The pain may be localized to the low back, sacroiliac, and lumbosacral joints; may refer to the buttocks and legs; and may involve the upper back. Unresolved back and pelvic joint pain in pregnancy can lead to chronic back and pelvic pain years postpartum.

Etiology
- Misalignments of the lumbosacral spine
- Pelvic and lumbosacral instability as a result of ligamentous laxity caused by the hormones of pregnancy
- Sacroiliac joint dysfunction
- Pubic symphysis separation
- Coccydynia
- Diastasis recti abdominis
- Posturally induced strain to localized segments of the lumbar spine, posterior musculature, and ligaments
- Lumbar and lumbosacral facet imbrication and inflammation as a result of the posterior shift in weight bearing necessitated by the increased abdominal girth
- Referred pain from trigger points in the posterior and anterior musculature
- Referred pain from strained uterine ligaments
- Fetal positioning
- Prolonged standing or sitting
- Wearing high-heeled shoes
- Insufficient back support while seated or lying down

Management
- Avoid contributing factors
- Assess and correct for sacroiliac, sacrococcygeal, symphysis pubis, and lumbosacral misalignments
- Use a sacroiliac belt
- Assess and treat hypertonicity, strain, and trigger points in the muscles and ligaments of the pelvis
- Make postural modifications

- Create individualized prescription of home exercises, including corrective exercises for pelvic misalignments, posture, and body mechanics training

Pain referral sights of uterine ligaments[*].

Broad ligaments—low back, buttock, and sciatica-like pain, especially in the sixth month and disappearing by the seventh and eighth months

Round ligaments—one-sided diagonal pain from the top of the uterus to the groin; more common in the second trimester

Sacrouterine ligaments—achy pain just lateral to or beneath the sacrum, primarily in the third trimester; pain in one or both buttocks

Morning Sickness

Morning sickness is a sensation of queasiness, nausea, and vomiting experienced by as many as 70% of women during the first trimester of pregnancy.

Etiology. The actual cause of morning sickness is unknown. Proposed causes include the following:

- Rising progesterone levels causing systemic muscle relaxation and slowing down the peristaltic motions of the digestive tract, causing slow elimination and an excess of stomach acids
- Rising levels of HCG
- Enhanced sense of smell

Technical Note

Severe morning sickness (hyperemesis gravidarum) is a serious medical condition that can result in dehydration, weight loss, and nutritional deficiencies.

Management

- Manage lifestyle
- Add fresh ginger to foods
- Drink ginger root tea

---

[*]From Osborne-Sheets C: *Pre and perinatal massage therapy: A comprehensive practitioner's guide to pregnancy, labor, postpartum*, 1st ed, San Diego, 1998, Body Therapy Associates.

- Eat several small meals during the day
- Keep hydrated
- Avoid strong food smells
- Eat crackers before getting out of bed in the morning
- Eat foods rich in vitamin B_6 such as nuts and legumes
- Take Vitamin B_6 supplement, up to 100 mg daily
- Apply acupressure to PC-6, which is located between the most lateral two tendons on the anterior surface of the forearm (i.e., the flexor carpi radialis and the palmaris longus tendons 2 inches proximal to the wrist crease). Deep rhythmic thumb or fingertip pressure is applied four times a day for 10 minutes each time.
- Perform generalized relaxation massage as tolerated
- Perform full spine assessment and manipulation with emphasis at C1 to influence the vagus nerve and enhance production of the food absorption hormones

Preeclampsia or Toxemia of Pregnancy

Preeclampsia is a condition marked by edema, elevated blood pressure, and abnormal protein in the urine during pregnancy. True preeclampsia occurs after the twentieth week of gestation.

- Preeclampsia occurs in approximately 7% of births.
- Eclampsia is severe and may result in seizure and coma.

Etiology
- Unknown

Signs and Symptoms
- Rapid weight gain from fluid retention—5 to 10 lb within 1 week
- Prominent swelling of the hands, face, and legs
- Severe headaches
- Blurred vision
- Edema

Fetal complications as a result of preeclampsia include inadequate fetal growth, premature labor, and fetal distress during labor.

Management. There is no known treatment for preeclampsia. Standard interventions include the following:

- Close monitoring
- Early delivery—preeclampsia resolves following the birth

- Hospitalization to control the blood pressure
- Bed rest—lying on the left side

Prevention. Studies have shown that expectant mothers who do not get enough riboflavin (vitamin B$_2$) are at increased risk for preeclampsia.

There have been anecdotal reports that chiropractic spinal manipulation may normalize blood pressure in some cases of preeclampsia.

Commentary

Michel Odent, author of *Birth Reborn*, states that there are no studies to suggest that bed rest is in fact of benefit in preventing or delaying premature labor, a primary concern of preeclampsia. Furthermore, he maintains that prolonged immobilization may lead to fetal sensory deprivation by limiting input to the vestibular organ, the inner part of the ear, which processes proprioceptive responses. In addition, Odent postulates that the vestibular organ possibly affects the fetus's orientation in utero, and deficiencies in its function might result in breech or shoulder presentations.

Premature Contractions

- Premature contractions are caused by a myriad of factors, some of which are life threatening and require crisis management, others of which are amenable to more conservative management protocols. Patients with premature contractions should first consult with their midwife or obstetrician. Premature contractions that are occurring in rapid succession warrant immediate medical attention.
- Dehydration, structural imbalance, and tipped uterus are common causes for premature contractions and are amenable to conservative management.

Technical Note

Risk factors for preterm labor include the following:
- Previous preterm birth
- Multiple pregnancy
- Incompetent cervix

- Uterine abnormalities
- Urinary tract infections
- Vaginal infections, commonly bacterial vaginosis
- Uterine exposure to diethylstilbestrol (DES)
- Diabetes
- Hypertension
- Thrombophilia and other clotting disorders
- Young maternal age
- Low prepregnancy weight
- Low weekly weight gain
- Nulliparity
- History of three or more abortions
- Late or no prenatal care
- Lifestyle factors such as smoking, drinking alcohol, and using illegal drugs
- Psychosocial factors such as stress, poverty, and lack of social support
- Domestic violence, including physical, sexual, or emotional abuse
- Short time period (less than 6 to 9 months) between pregnancies

---

Pubic Diastases (Symphysis Pubis Pain)

Symphysis pubis pain is pain in the pelvic girdle, deep groin, or medial thigh caused by a shift in the pubic and pelvic bones, most commonly occurring in pregnancy or in the postpartum period.

Etiology. As pregnancy progresses and systemic levels of oxytocin and relaxin increase, the fibrocartilaginous ligaments at the symphysis pubis become increasingly lax. This increase in laxity predisposes to misalignment of the bony structures of the pelvis.

Signs and symptoms

- Gradually increasing pelvic and low back pain as pregnancy progresses
- Sciatica
- Moderate to severe pain directly over the symphysis pubis
- Pain deep in the groin or lower abdomen
- Pain with fundal height assessment
- Lower abdominal, pelvic, or pubic pain that occurs when

- Climbing stairs
- Getting in and out of an automobile
- Engaging in sexual activity
- Putting on underwear
- Walking
- Moderate to severe pain over the pubic bone when turning over in bed or sleeping on the side
- Pain in the lower abdomen over the round ligament
- Clicking or popping in the area of the symphysis pubis with locomotion

Diagnosis

- Signs and symptoms
- Biomechanical assessment of the pelvic girdle and surrounding musculature
- Measurement of width of the symphysis by x-ray or real-time ultrasound

Management

Lifestyle factors

- An ice pack placed over the site of pain
- Sleeping with a pillow between the knees provides some stability to the pelvis
- Enlisting a partner to support the hips by holding them on either side when turning in bed
- Standing for prolonged periods should be limited and effort to ensure the even distribution of weight to both feet is necessary
- Dressing in the seated position, especially when it is necessary to wear clothing that requires inserting one leg at a time
- Skirts and dresses should be worn instead of pants and pulled down from the top rather than up from the bottom
- Maternity support belts may be useful
- Swinging the legs as a unit may be helpful when entering or exiting cars
- Remaining well hydrated by drinking water regularly

Manipulation

- Pelvic manipulation is very helpful in this condition.
- Direct adjustment to realign the symphysis pubis often is necessary.

Physical therapy

- Instruction in self-realignment of pelvic joints
- Pelvic floor muscle activation during transitional movements

- Instruction in compensatory movement strategies
- Core muscle strengthening
- Sacroiliac belt

Massage

- Massage to the low back muscles and over the round ligament

Medications

- Anti-inflammatory medication
- Pain killers
- Steroid injections

Prevention

Biomechanical assessment and realignment of the pelvis during pregnancy. This is especially critical in individuals who have a prior history of pelvic misalignments or low back pain.

Rhesus Factor

The Rh factor is found in the blood of 85% of white individuals and 95% of black individuals. People who have Rh factor are known as Rh positive. Those who do not are Rh negative. Being Rh negative has no impact on the individual's general health; however, when the mother is Rh negative and the father and the baby are both Rh positive, Rh disease (also known as hemolytic disease of the newborn) may occur.

The Rh-positive blood inherited from the father may leak into the mother's circulation during pregnancy, but more commonly during delivery. The mother who is Rh negative makes Rh-positive antibodies; this can hurt subsequent pregnancies because the antibodies can cross the placenta and destroy some of the fetal red blood cells, producing anemia, which can lead to serious and even fatal brain damage.

Management. Rh disease is increasingly rare because Rh-negative mothers are given the drug RhoGAM at 28 weeks of gestation and immediately postpartum, and this prevents the formation of antibodies in an Rh-negative mother. Rh-positive mothers do not have to worry, even if the father is Rh negative. Rh blood typing and testing currently are performed routinely at the first visit. If the mother is Rh positive, there is no cause for concern. If, however, the mother is Rh negative, the father should be checked. If he also is Rh negative, there is no concern, because the baby will be Rh negative and there is no risk of antibody production. If the father is Rh positive, there is susceptibility for disease and the test will be repeated to check for antibodies in the sixth and eighth months and at delivery. Amniocentesis may be performed to check for bilirubin, which is released into the amniotic fluid if and when the fetal blood cells are broken down by maternal Rh antibodies.

Snoring

Etiology. The increased blood flow into the mucous membranes causes swelling, which restricts airflow and causes snoring.
Management. Sleeping on the side instead of on the back prevents the tongue and soft palate from resting against the back of the throat and further blocking the airways.

Anecdotal reports suggest that wearing a nasal strip might be helpful.

Spontaneous Abortion (Miscarriage)

Spontaneous abortion, also known as *miscarriage,* is the loss of the pregnancy within the first 20 weeks of gestation.
Etiology. There are a myriad of postulated causes for miscarriage, including the following:
- Chromosome abnormalities in the sperm or egg
- Maternal factors such as diabetes, smoking, alcohol use, age over 35 years, anatomic defects of the uterus
- Luteal phase defects
- Unknown
Signs and symptoms
- Vaginal bleeding or spotting
- Severe, persistent headaches
- Prolonged vomiting, severe enough to prevent adequate intake of liquids
- Blurred vision or spots before the eyes
- Fever and chills not accompanied by a cold
- Sudden intense or continual abdominal pains and cramping
- Sudden gush of fluid from the vagina

- Sudden swelling of hands, feet, and ankles
- Frequent burning urination
- Pronounced decrease in fetal movement

Management
- Assessments and interventions for the contributing factors
- Luteal phase defect (also known as inadequate progesterone) is diagnosed by endometrial biopsy and treated in subsequent pregnancies with progesterone vaginal suppositories or progesterone creams.

Thoracic Outlet Syndrome

Thoracic outlet syndrome is pain, numbness, and tingling either in a glovelike distribution or following a specific dermatomal pattern in the hand and along the arm.

Etiology
- Postural compromise as the abdominal girth and breasts enlarge
- Edema

Management
- Provide trigger point therapy to the pectoralis and scalene muscles
- Assess and manipulate the cervicothoracic spine as warranted
- Stretch and strengthen the anterior, middle, and posterior scalene muscles
- Assess and modify postural inadequacies
- Perform rehabilitative exercises
- Apply physiotherapy modalities

Tipped Uterus

A tipped uterus is a uterus that tips forward in a pelvic cavity that typically has endured prior undiagnosed or untreated trauma. The added pressure and weight of the amniotic fluid and the growing baby apply stress to the unstable sacral segments, causing them to buckle.

Technical Note

The uterus is anchored by several ligaments that must evenly distribute the tension for maximum balance. If the ligaments on the anterior surface of the uterus contract more than those in the back, the uterus is pulled forward. Pressure on the nerves and arteries that supply the muscles of the groin and upper thigh may result, and movement, especially walking, is compromised. Extreme cervical pressure occurs, and premature labor may result.

Management
• Buckled sacrum maneuver (see Appendix)

Clinical Pearl

"My feet flew out from underneath me before I fell on my bottom" is a typical scenario elicited in the prior history from a woman with premature labor that may be caused by a "buckled sacrum."

Urinary Frequency/Urgency

Etiology
• Increased pressure on the bladder as the size of the uterus increases
• Urinary tract or bladder infection

Management
• Identify and treat any pathogens. The most common are bacterial vaginosis and candidiasis.
• Assess for contributing factors, including diet.
• Perform pelvic floor muscle (Kegel) exercises (see Appendix).

Urinary Stress Incontinence

Etiology. Muscles of the pelvic floor may become overstretched and weakened in pregnancy. Approximately 33% of women report urinary incontinence in pregnancy.

Clinical Pearl

Women with incontinence during pregnancy are more likely to suffer long-term symptoms of urinary incontinence.

Management
• Pelvic floor muscle training in pregnancy, which also has been shown to reduce the risk of urinary incontinence postpartum
• See Chapter 19 Clinical notes

Diagnostic Tests during Pregnancy

- Fundal height
- Blood pressure
- Papanicolaou (Pap) smears to rule out cervical cancer and sexually transmitted diseases and a vaginal culture to rule out streptococcus B infection
- Urinalysis to rule out infections, elevated sugars, and proteins
- Ultrasound to evaluate the fetus at various stages of development
- Weight gain

Blood Tests—First Trimester

- Blood type and antibody screen, including Rh factor
- Hematocrit and hemoglobin to rule out anemia
- Hepatitis B virus
- Human immunodeficiency virus (HIV)
- Rubella
- Syphilis

Blood Tests—Second and Third Trimesters

- Hematocrit and hemoglobin to rule out anemia
- Glucose tolerance test to screen for gestational diabetes

Specialized Tests

Maternal alpha-fetoprotein (AFP) or expanded alpha-fetoprotein testing, which includes estriol and HCG to screen for neural tube defects, Down syndrome, and other chromosome abnormalities. False-positive results are not uncommon.

Amniocentesis

- Evaluation for birth defects is performed at 16 to 18 weeks of gestation. May be recommended if either parent has a disease with genetic components, if the parents have a child who has a genetic component, or if the mother is over 35.
- Evaluation for fetal maturity when repeat cesarean section is planned. This is performed at 38 to 39 weeks of gestation.

- Evaluation for fetal maturity in high-risk pregnancies, such as with high blood pressure, diabetes, Rh disease, and inadequate fetal growth; and when the mother is overdue by more than 2 weeks. The risk of the procedure's causing miscarriage is approximately 0.5% to 2%.

NUTRITION AND PREGNANCY

- At no other time are the woman's nutritional needs more important. Adequate intake of fresh fruits, whole grains, vegetables, proteins, calcium, vitamin A, vitamin D, iron, and folic acid are critical. A prenatal multivitamin is necessary for most women.
- Increased dose of folic acid is recommended preconceptually to prevent open neural tube defects.

Clinical Pearl
- *Vegetarian diets may manifest deficiencies in protein, iodine, iron, and folate.*
- *Iodized salt is recommended over sea salt to ensure proper functioning of the thyroid gland.*
- *Tofu is an excellent source of protein for the vegetarian, but it may contain bacteria. Unpackaged tofu should not be eaten in pregnancy, and packaged tofu should be cooked to an internal temperature of 160° F.*

Weight Gain in Pregnancy

Emphasis should be placed on the quality of the diet, rather than the amount of weight gained; however, during the second half of the pregnancy, caloric intake should increase by about 10%.

A 20 to 30 lb weight gain generally is recommended. Actual weight gain is patient specific because some women can gain more and still maintain a healthy pregnancy.

Average gain in pregnancy
Baby: 7 to 8 lb
Placenta: 1.5 lb
Amniotic fluid: 2 lb
Uterus: 2 lb
Breasts: 1 to 1.5 lb

Blood: 3 to 4 lb
Fluid retained in body tissues: 2 to 3 lb
Maternal stores (fat, protein) not in nutrients: 3.5 to 6 lb
Total: 22 to 28 lb

EXERCISE AND PREGNANCY

- Exercise helps to prepare a woman's body for labor and delivery, and when done in moderation poses no danger to mother or baby. Exercise may help with constipation, backache, edema, and poor posture.
- Pregnancy is not the time to begin a strenuous exercise program.
- Activities that may result in decreased oxygen to the fetus should be avoided. These include strenuous activity, scuba diving, sprinting, competitive exercise, high-altitude training, and contact sports. In addition, activities where water can be forced into the vagina should be avoided, including water skiing and surfing. Exercise should be avoided or minimized in hot, humid weather. Elevated body temperatures have been linked to birth defects.
- To avoid the risk of dehydration, drinking plenty of fluids while exercising is recommended.

FETAL DEVELOPMENTS

- *First trimester (first to third months).* Fetal developments include formation of the head, brain, spine, heart, body, limbs, and sex organs. Caution about drugs and chemicals is warranted in this trimester, because drugs and chemicals may cross the placenta and influence the development of the fetus.
- *Second trimester (fourth to sixth months).* Fetal developments include maturation of the circulatory system and skeletal movements. Assessing the mother's daily activities to ensure frequent rest is recommended.
- *Third trimester (seventh to ninth months).* This is a period of rapid fetal growth. The fetus multiplies its weight three to four times. It is important to ensure that the mother remains well hydrated and that protein intake is adequate.

29

Pregnancy—Labor and Delivery

PREGNANCY—LABOR

There are three stages of labor and delivery:
- The first stage is the time of dilation of the cervix and includes the early, active, and transition phases. The early phase manifests at 3 to 4 cm of dilation and is the most comfortable of the three stages; the active phase manifests at approximately 4 to 7 cm of dilation, and the contractions become more intense. Breathing techniques may be useful. The phase of transition manifests at approximately 8 to 10 cm of dilation, and the pain and pressure are most intense.
- The second stage begins when the cervix is completely dilated and ends when the baby is born. It typically averages 20 minutes to 1 hour but can last for several hours. It is marked by a tremendous urge to bear down and push the baby out.
- The third stage is delivery of the afterbirth, or placenta, and usually occurs within 30 minutes after the birth.

LABOR INDUCTION

Procedures to induce labor in women who are considerably past the due date include the following:
- Lifestyle factors
- Nipple stimulation with a rough-textured face towel
- Massage—muscle stripping techniques applied to the adductors
- Acupressure—bone-to-bone pressure to the uterus and ovary zones at the midpoint of the medial and lateral calcaneus, respectively

- Acupuncture—acupuncture points that commonly are needled to promote uterine contractions include the following:
  - Spleen 6, four client finger widths proximal to the malleolus along the medial tibial border
  - Kidney 3, on the superior border and just posterior to the medial malleolus
  - Liver 3, at the proximal border of the first and second metatarsal bones
  - Hoku hand point, at the junction of the thumb and index finger
- Spinal and pelvic manipulation
- Medications
  - Pitocin (the hormone oxytocin) typically given intravenously
  - Prostaglandin gels or vaginal inserts such as Cervidil, which soften and dilate the cervix
- Medical procedures
  - Amniotomy, in which the amniotic sac is ruptured
  - "Stripping the membrane," in which the membrane that connects the amniotic sac to the uterine wall is stripped; this causes the release of prostaglandins, which help to prepare the cervix for delivery and may induce contractions

BACK LABOR

Etiology

One of the causes of back labor is the baby's exiting in the occiput posterior position. The front of the baby's head is turned toward the pubic bone and the back of the head toward the sacrum. The converse is the ideal. The back of the head against the sacrum puts pressure on the parasympathetic nerves exiting the sacral foramen, and this can be very painful for the mother.

Management

Comfort measures:
- Pressure applied to the sacrum, usually with the fists of the partner
- Warm poultices applied to the low back

- Craniosacral therapy
- Respiratory and pelvic diaphragm release techniques
- The side-lying maneuver—see Appendix

30

Pregnancy—Postpartum

WHAT IS IT?

In a process called *involution*, which lasts about 6 weeks, the uterus returns to its normal size. The process occurs in a series of uterine contractions, often termed *afterpains*. The multiparous woman may experience more contractions than the primiparous woman because the uterus tends to be a little more lax. Involution is under the control of oxytocin, the same hormone that causes the milk to "let down."

Conditions affiliated with the postpartum include the following:
- Abdominal laxity
- Breast filling
- Breast pain
- Cesarean management
- Constipation
- Diabetes
- Itching from the stitches
- Loss of bladder sensitivity
- Nipple pain
- Postpartum depression
- Sore perineum
- Vaginal drainage
- Weight loss

ABDOMINAL LAXITY

Etiology

A certain degree of abdominal laxity is expected in the postpartum and may result in diastasis recti abdominis.

Management

To minimize this possibility, and to restore the abdominal girth to its regular tone, abdominal exercises are recommended, beginning with abdominal breathing and followed carefully and cautiously by abdominal isometrics, pelvic rocking, and curl-ups. Activation of the transverse abdominis muscle is recommended to initiate abdominal muscle recovery.

FILLING OF THE BREASTS
Etiology

The presence of the infant at the nipple is a stimulus to the anterior pituitary gland to release prolactin. Prolactin is responsible for initiating milk production. When the infant begins to suckle, the suckling effect stimulates the neurohypophysis to release oxytocin. Oxytocin causes contraction of the myoepithelial cells that line the alveoli, propelling the fluid forward into the lactiferous ducts behind the areola. The result is the let-down reflex, often described as the filling of the breasts. The woman simultaneously may experience contraction of the uterus.

Technical Note

The initial fluid that the infant gets from the breast is colostrum, which is valuable in proteins, minerals, antibodies and other immune factors. Colostrum enables the infant to eliminate any meconium that is in the gastrointestinal tract as a result of the birth and eliminate excess bilirubin.

Management

• Comfort measures

BREAST PAIN
Etiology

The "coming in" of the milk occurs on or about the third day and results in marked engorgement of the breasts. This often is accompanied by pain, tenderness, or throbbing of the breasts and sometimes a mild fever.

Management

- Frequent nursing and the use of a supportive bra.
- Reassurance—the discomfort commonly resolves in 7 to 10 days once mother and baby are on a regular nursing schedule.
- If the mother does not plan to nurse, she should wear a supportive bra and avoid expressing any milk, use ice therapies for relief, and pain medications as prescribed.

CESAREAN SECTION

Management

- Wound and scar management
- Rehabilitation
- Bracing body mechanics
- No lifting over 15 lb; no heavy household duties; avoid any activities that cause pain

CONSTIPATION

Etiology

The first bowel movement may not occur until a few days after delivery, and constipation is common. The mother's fear of exerting pressure as a result of soreness in the perineal region, hemorrhoids, healing episiotomy scars, sluggish intestinal peristaltic action, and lax abdominal muscles all contribute to constipation.

Management

If the mother has not returned to normal bowel functioning by the third day, stool softeners or laxatives may be recommended. She should be encouraged to increase fiber and water as tolerated and to take short walks to facilitate motion.

DIABETES

Appropriate follow-up for all patients diagnosed with gestational diabetes includes the following:

- Recommend all diabetes prevention strategies.
- A postpartum glucose tolerance test should be performed to determine risk of developing type 2 diabetes.

- The patient should be screened for type 2 diabetes yearly or every 3 years, depending on the results of the initial postpartum tests.

ITCHING FROM EPISIOTOMY STITCHES
Management

This will resolve spontaneously, but the mother can be advised to sit on an inflatable doughnut pillow and to use cold compresses.

LOSS OF BLADDER SENSITIVITY

The early postpartum is a period of diuresis as the excess fluid accumulated during the pregnancy is eliminated.

Management

- The mother should be reminded to be attentive to cues to urinate because there might be a slight loss of bladder sensitivity to fluid pressure as a result of the trauma exerted during the birth process.
- See Chapter 19.

NIPPLE PAIN

The infant's suckling and suckling techniques can result in nipple pain.

Management

- Preparing the nipple by rubbing with a rough-textured towel in the weeks approaching the due date
- In the postpartum, expressing some of the milk immediately before nursing may allow the infant to find the nipple more easily
- Applying cold compress on the breasts and nipples

POSTPARTUM DEPRESSION

As many as 80% of women experience the postpartum blues, which is a brief period during which women are tearful and sensitive. Postpartum blues should resolve within 1 to 2 weeks.

Postpartum depression may occur immediately or several months after the birth and can last for days, weeks, months and, in some cases, years. As many as 14% of women develop postpartum depression. Postpartum depression is thought to result from the rapidly fluctuating internal (hormonal) and external (physical) environment.

Management

Lifestyle
- Managing the psychosocial issues, which might involve
  - Obtaining experienced help for baby care
  - Getting plenty of rest and sleep
  - Finding a support system
- Stress management
- Exercise
- Foot reflexology for relaxation

Vitamins, minerals, and herbs
- St. John's wort standardized to contain 0.3% hypericum is proven useful in the management of depression
- Progesterone cream may be recommended

Medications
- Avoid premature use of hormonal birth control methods
- Consider antidepressants such as Prozac, if necessary

Counseling
- Talk therapy with a trained professional may be helpful.

A plethora of additional symptoms have been linked to the postpartum. These include, but are not limited to, impaired mother-infant interactions, bipolar disorders, posttraumatic stress disorder, back pain, pelvic pain, postpartum anxiety disorders, frequent headaches, various forms of psychosis, dyspareunia, stress incontinence, anemia, and hemorrhoids. The author refers the reader to the Diagnostic and Statistical Manual of Mental Disorders (DSM) guidelines on postpartum conditions for additional information on most of these conditions.

SORE PERINEUM

As a result of the tremendous stretching by the perineum, there is some soreness after the birth, even if an episiotomy has not been performed.

Management

- Reinstitute pelvic floor muscle (Kegel) exercises as soon as possible.
- Sit meditation style, if tolerated, to place the pressure evenly on the ischial tuberosities, instead of on the perineum.
- Wash the vaginal area regularly with warm water. A squeeze bottle can be used.
- Apply cold packs to the perineum.
- Take sitz baths, which may be helpful.

VAGINAL DRAINAGE

Vaginal drainage, or lochia, occurs for the first few days after childbirth but may be plentiful for 2 to 3 weeks and may last for up to 6 weeks. This process, which feels to many women like a heavy menstrual period, enables the endometrium to heal by sloughing off the superficial layer of cells and necrotic tissue from the placental site, with concurrent regrowth of healthy new epithelium. The lochia changes in color from red or pink to brown or yellow and eventually to whitish.

Management

- Comfort measures

  Women who fear this blood loss can be reminded that the body has taken on a greater volume of blood during pregnancy.

WEIGHT LOSS

The expulsion of the uterine contents results in about a 10 to 12 lb weight loss. Diuresis and diaphoresis result in the loss of an additional 5 lb. The increased caloric utilization affiliated with nursing (milk production) typically results in additional weight loss over the subsequent months.

CLINICAL NOTES

Postpartum—Nutrition Needs

- Increase hydration
- Consume more nutrients

It is recommended that the postpartum woman should eat more of most nutrients than she consumed during pregnancy. The body requires more energy to produce milk, and the milk requires substantial calories. To produce 1 quart of milk per day when breast-feeding, the mother must consume about 900 extra calories daily. No nourishing foods need to be eliminated from the diet.

Technical Note

Some foods ingested by the mother may have undesirable effects on the infant. These include the following:

- Chocolate, which may have a laxative effect
- Broccoli, brussels sprouts, cabbage, dried beans, and cauliflower, which may create gas
- Spicy foods, which may flavor the milk or cause gas pains

Clinical Pearl

Brown spots on fairer-skinned women or white spots on darker-skinned women (i.e., the "mask of pregnancy" or "pregnancy cap") that do not disappear within a month after delivery might indicate folic acid deficiency. Supplementation with 5 mg of folic acid per meal should restore normal skin tone within 2 to 3 weeks.

31

Premature Ovarian Failure

WHAT IS IT?

Premature ovarian failure (POF) is the appearance of menopausal symptoms in women younger than age 40. Women in POF frequently exhibit amenorrhea, hypoestrogenism, and elevated serum gonadotropin levels.

Technical Note

The hypothalamic-pituitary-ovarian axis is regulated by several hormones, including estradiol, the androgens, and inhibins, which are secreted by the ovarian follicles. One dominant follicle typically matures with each cycle; however, its maturation is dependent on the development of thousands of nondominant follicles. Conditions resulting from a reduction in the numbers of these nondominant follicles often manifest with a decline of the ovarian hormones, subsequent elevation of the pituitary hormones, and an overall disruption of the hypothalamic-pituitary-ovarian axis.

WHO GETS IT?

Premature ovarian failure can occur only in women under age 40. If ovarian failure occurs over age 40, it is considered to be a normal menopausal state. Approximately 1% of women experience menopause before age 40.

ETIOLOGY

POF can be spontaneous or iatrogenically induced.

- Iatrogenic ovarian failure is caused by follicular developmental arrest and follicular depletion, which is due to damage to the granulosa cells and the oocytes. In addition, interstitial fibrosis and hyalinization of blood vessels may occur.
- Spontaneous ovarian failure is presumed to fall into two broad categories:
  - Follicular depletion as a result of a depleted follicle reserve, a low initial number of follicles, or an accelerated rate of follicle atresia.
  - Follicle dysfunction as a result of failure to grow and ovulate while under the influence of otherwise normally functioning endocrine systems. An example would be a follicle that, instead of progressing to a normal ovulation, is inappropriately luteinized and persists as a cyst.

Iatrogenic Causes

- Bilateral oophorectomy
- Chemotherapy
- Radiation therapy
- Bone marrow transplant
- Treatment with busulfan

The ovarian cells are sensitive tissues that respond adversely to systemic treatments such as chemotherapy, radiation therapy, gonadal irritation, and various forms of cancer therapy. Following bone marrow transplant and therapy with busulfan, the majority of women develop ovarian failure.

Spontaneous Causes

- Cleaning solvents. There is evidence that some women have developed premature ovarian failure after exposure to cleaning solvents containing the agent 2-bromopropane. In some cases the ovaries recover spontaneously and regular menstrual cycles may ensue, although reduced fertility and increased serum follicle-stimulating hormone (FSH) levels may persist.
- Genetic defects involving the X chromosome or autosomes have been implicated as plausible causes for POF. X chromosome genes are involved in regulating female fertility.

Evidence suggests that half of the patients with partial deletions of the short arm of the X chromosome have amenorrhea. Other chromosomal aberrations that have been implicated in premature ovarian failure include the following:

- Trisomy 13 and 18 are associated with ovarian dysgenesis and failure.
- 46 XX is affiliated with gonadal dysgenesis.
- Abnormalities of the forkhead transcription factor gene located on chromosome 3q22–23 are known to result in resistant ovaries (ovaries contain many follicles that do not develop) and subsequent ovarian depletion.
- Enzyme deficiencies have been affiliated with ovarian failure, including cholesterol desmolase deficiency, which results in lipid-filled adrenals and a lack of ovarian function; 17α-hydroxylase deficiency, which results in ovarian failure from impaired ovarian and adrenal hormone synthesis; deficiency of the 17–20 desmolase enzyme, a part of the 17α-hydroxylase cytochrome P450 complex, which results in low serum estrogens, high gonadotropins, enlarged ovaries with multiple cysts, and amenorrhea; and deficiency of the aromatase enzyme, needed for synthesis of estrogen and found in adipose tissues, which has been demonstrated to result in a lack of pubertal development, high serum gonadotropin levels, and multiple ovarian cysts.
- Autoimmune disorders include adrenal autoimmunity, Addison's disease, antiovarian antibodies, type 1 diabetes, Hashimoto's thyroiditis with or without hypothyroidism, lupus, rheumatoid arthritis, and Sjogren's syndrome.
- Infections such as mumps, malaria, and varicella have been noted in women with POF; however, a direct cause-and-effect relationship has not been established.

DIAGNOSIS

Detailed History

- Menstrual history, including last spontaneous menstrual cycle, time of menarche, and previous menstrual patterns
- History of pelvic surgeries, radiation therapy, or chemotherapy
- Prior exposure to toxic environmental agents
- History of infection
- Symptoms of adrenal insufficiency, including

- Orthostatic hypotension
- Skin hyperpigmentation
- Unexplained weakness
- Salt craving
- Abdominal pain
- Anorexia
- Symptoms of hypothyroidism
- Family history of POF
- Family history of male mental retardation
- Family history of autoimmune disorders

Clinical Pearl

The history of a patient with POF can be variable, depending on the pathogenesis. In cases of spontaneous ovarian failure, the typical scenario is a sudden onset of amenorrhea, usually after discontinuation of oral contraceptives or after a pregnancy. In as many as 50% of cases, a long history of oligomenorrhea and polymenorrhea, with or without menopausal symptoms, is present. In 10% of the affected women, POF manifests as primary amenorrhea. Occasionally, menopausal symptoms appear before the menses have stopped.

Physical Examination

- Signs of hypoestrogenism
- Presence/absence of palpable ovaries
- Physical signs of Turner's syndrome or other genetic syndromes, including
  - Short stature
  - Webbed neck
  - Low position of the ears
  - Low posterior hairline
  - Cubitus valgus
  - Shield chest
  - Short IV and V metacarpals
- Signs of autoimmune diseases, Addison's disease, and hypothyroidism

Tests

- Pregnancy test
- FSH, luteinizing hormone (LH), estradiol

- Two FSH levels in the menopausal range of over 40 mIU/ml measured at least 1 month apart are diagnostic of POF
- LH is typically elevated
- Estradiol levels are low

Technical Note

In some cases, women with POF have spontaneous follicular activity, which may result in erroneous laboratory results. If the index of suspicion for POF is high, the tests are repeated within a couple of months.

- Additional testing may include the following:
  - Standard blood chemistry—fasting glucose, electrolytes, and creatinine
  - Karyotyping
  - Test for fragile X chromosome (*FMR1* premutation)
  - Thyroid-stimulating hormone (TSH)
  - Antithyroid peroxidase antibody
  - Serum adrenal antibodies
  - Screen for other autoimmune disorders
  - Bone density by dual-energy x-ray absorptiometry (DEXA) scan
  - Screen and test for exposure to environmental and other toxins
  - Ovarian biopsy and ultrasound are not recommended in this diagnostic evaluation

Differential Diagnosis

Differential diagnosis should include the following:
- Pregnancy
- Secondary ovarian failure attributable to factors such as eating disorders and intense exercise
- Systemic diseases
- Medications
- Polycystic ovary syndrome (PCOS)
- Outflow tract abnormalities

Signs and Symptoms

- Amenorrhea before age 40
- Early onset of menopausal-like symptoms as a result of a prolonged hypoestrogenic state, including
  - Hot flashes
  - Sweats
  - Vaginal dryness and atrophic vaginitis
  - Irritability
  - Symptoms of hypothyroidism, such as dry eyes, dry skin, and generalized fatigue
- Dyspareunia
- Decreased libido

Other symptoms caused by prolonged hypoestrogenism include osteoporosis and a higher risk for cardiovascular disease.

MANAGEMENT

There is no proven cure for infertile patients with premature ovarian failure. Assisted conception with donated oocytes and hormonal therapy are treatments most commonly used. Embryo, ovarian tissue or oocyte cryopreservation may be recommended in cases in which ovarian failure is anticipated, such as when chemotherapy, radiation therapy, and other cancer treatments are necessary.

Treatments are designed to manage for the accelerated menopausal state and hypoandrogenism and include the following:

- Oral contraceptives
- Hormonal replacement therapy in an age-related dose
- TSH and adrenal antibodies
- Short-term androgen replacement for women with persistent fatigue and low libido
- DEXA bone density scan; supplementation with calcium, magnesium, vitamin D, vitamin K, and trace minerals; and weight-bearing exercises to prevent osteoporosis
- Specific medications for osteoporosis prevention and management
- Psychologic evaluation and counseling for the grief and loss associated with a diagnosis of POF

Technical Note

Anecdotal reports have suggested that high-dose, long-term prednisone therapy may be useful in treating autoimmune ovarian failure. However, when used in high doses for long periods of time, prednisone has substantial side effects, including aseptic necrosis of bone.

Herbs and Adaptogens

Rhodiola rosea has been shown to restore menses in women when given at a dose of 100 mg extract orally twice a day for 2 weeks, or 1 ml rhodosin intramuscularly for 10 days. In a study of 40 women given these dosages, menses was restored in 25, and pregnancy ensued in 11. In some subjects the treatment cycle was repeated two to four times. Furthermore, there is evidence that *Rhodiola rosea* extract shows strong estrogen-binding properties.

- Endocrine system detoxification:
  - Whole-foods diet
  - Flaxseed 1 to 2 tablespoons per day
  - Soy 1 to 2 servings per day
  - Liver support, including milk thistle, dandelion root, beet root, and burdock root
  - Black cohosh 40 mg of the standardized extract twice daily
  - Maca root 2 g/day
  - Vitex 40 drops of the tincture daily or 20 mg of standardized extract daily
  - Partridge berry
  - *Rhodiola* 200 mg/day
  - Yarrow 2 tsp/day
  - Calcium 500 mg twice daily
  - Vitamin D 1000 IU daily
  - Trace minerals

Technical Note

The risk of osteoporosis is high in patients with POF. It is imperative that hormones be used if alternative methods of management do not result in the restoration of normal monthly cycles within 6 months.

Technical Note

Premature ovarian failure caused by inappropriate regulatory signals (hypothalamic or pituitary pathology) is secondary ovarian failure. Premature ovarian failure as a result of a pathologic process directly affecting the ovaries (e.g., chemotherapy, irradiation, autoimmunity, chromosomal abnormalities) is primary ovarian failure.

- A means of distinguishing between the two conditions is to measure serum FSH and LH levels, which will be elevated in primary ovarian failure and low or normal in secondary ovarian failure.
- Many women with POF retain intermittent ovarian function for many years, and, unlike women who are menopausal, pregnancies may occur spontaneously.

32

Premenstrual Syndrome (PMS)

WHAT IS IT?

Premenstrual syndrome (PMS) is an umbrella term for a broad range of symptoms that begin after ovulation, peak before menstruation, and diminish after menses.

WHO GETS IT?

Women in their menstruating years, most commonly women ages 25 to 40. Some studies suggest that 60% to 80% of women in the United States have some premenstrual symptoms.

ETIOLOGY

Proposed causes of PMS include the following:
- Alterations in the normal estrogen-to-progesterone ratios, with a preponderance of estrogen during the luteal phase
- Altered serotonin and dopamine levels
- Altered prostaglandin levels—the inflammatory prostaglandins dominating
- Vitamin and mineral insufficiencies—vitamin B_6 and magnesium commonly are identified as lacking
- Suboptimal liver function
- Suboptimal gastrointestinal function

SIGNS AND SYMPTOMS

- Irritability
- Mood swings

- Swelling of the abdomen, breasts, and ankles
- Restlessness
- Tension
- Depression
- Anxiety
- Sore and tender breasts
- Headaches
- Food cravings
- Weight gain
- Memory loss
- Decreased concentration and forgetfulness

PMS CLASSIFICATION

The Guy Abrahams PMS classification chart system identifies four subgroups:

- Premenstrual tension (PMT)
  - **PMT-A** (anxiety): marked by nervous tension, mood swings, irritability, anxiety, and insomnia
  - **PMT-C** (craving): marked by cravings for sugars and sweets, increased appetite, occasional episodes of arrhythmia, dizzy spells, fainting, and fatigue
  - **PMT-H** (hyperhydration): marked by weight gain (greater than 3 lb [1.4 kg]), swelling of the extremities, breast tenderness, and abdominal bloating
  - **PMT-D** (depression): marked by episodes of depression, forgetfulness, crying, and confusion

PMT-A, PMT-C, and PMT-H are thought to be caused in part by estrogen dominance; PMT-D is thought to be caused in part by fluctuations in mean blood progesterone.

Technical Note

Insulin resistance predisposes to estrogen dominance in part by increasing fat and, consequently, fat cell storage of estrogen.

DIAGNOSIS

- Signs and symptoms
- Daily record of symptoms for 2 to 3 months—symptoms are ranked from most distressing to least distressing.

- Timing of symptoms in relation to the menstrual cycle
- Thyroid hormone assessment
- Nutritional status assessment
- Comprehensive hormonal assay

A diagnosis of PMS can be made if there is a clear pattern of symptoms that begin after ovulation and resolve or subside with menses.

Premenstrual dysphoric disorder (PMDD) is a severe form of PMS, classified in the Diagnostic and Statistical Manual of Mental Disorders (DSM) as a psychiatric disorder. Some authorities suggest that all levels of PMS are best assessed and managed as psychologic or psychiatric disorders.

MANAGEMENT

Lifestyle Factors

- Regular moderate aerobic exercise
- Filtered drinking water (water from public drinking systems may contain estrogen and estrogen byproducts)
- Dietary intake of flaxseed, soy, and other fiber and lignan sources, which
  - Modulate estrogen levels by up-regulating the production of the sex hormone–binding globulins (SHBGs)
  - Populate selective receptor sites with less potent phyto-estrogens
  - Facilitate the elimination of (more potent) estrogens
  - Avoid/minimize red meat and dairy intake—these are sources of arachidonic acid, a precursor to the inflammatory prostaglandins
  - Minimize exposure to exogenous estrogens (xenoestrogens)—this includes environmental factors such as fuels and pesticides, dietary sources such as hormone-fattened cattle and livestock, and ancillary lifestyle factors such as microwaving in plastic containers
  - Minimize intake of refined sugars
  - Minimize alcohol intake, which interferes with some of the B vitamins, magnesium, and chromium
  - Limit caffeine, which can intensify anxiety

Technical Note

Estrogen is transported through the blood system bound to SHBGs. While bound, estrogen is unavailable to tissue.

Vitamins, Minerals, and Herbs

- Vitamin B_6 in a B complex up to 500 mg/day for 3 months facilitates the excretion of estrogen and estrogen byproducts and aids in the synthesis of anti-inflammatory prostaglandins. Doses less than 200 mg do not appear to offer benefit for PMS symptoms.
- Magnesium up to 400 mg/day aids with prostaglandin synthesis and red blood cell magnesium.
- Vitamin D studies have indicated that women with vitamin D intake of an average of 706 IU/day are at significantly lower risk for PMS than those with intake of 112 IU/day.
- Calcium. Women with an average of 1280 mg/day calcium intake from food are at lower PMS risk than those with lower intake of 529 mg/day.
- L-tryptophan. Women with PMDD who were given 6 g of L-tryptophan during the luteal phase noted improvements in dysphoria, mood swings, tension, and irritability.
- Herbs such as chaste tree berry *(Vitex agnus)* regulate the hypothalamic-pituitary axis by acting directly on the pituitary to stimulate luteinizing hormone (LH) secretion and inhibit follicle-stimulating hormone (FSH) secretion. This can result in an increase of progesterone, which decreases the estrogen-to-progesterone ratios in the premenstruum. Chaste berry in the form of *Vitex agnus* extract Ze 440, 20 mg per day, was shown to relieve symptoms of headache, breast tenderness, mood swings, and bloating (Schellenberg, 2001). Primary Symptoms of Mastodynia
- Gingko biloba (80 mg twice a day in the luteal phase) (Tamborini, 1993)
- Evening primrose oil 2 g daily in split doses; this is fat soluble and should be taken with meals
- Soy isoflavones 68 mg/day (Bryan, 2005)

Primary symptoms of depression. St. John's wort. Hypericum inhibits serotonin uptake and is useful where primary symptoms are depression. Dosage is up to 50% (6.2 mcg/ml) or 0.3% standardized extract.

Neurolymphatic Points for Symptom Relief

- Cramps/low back pain: upper edges of the pubic bone; L2–4 lamina
- Breast tenderness: fifth and sixth intercostal spaces; T5–7 lamina
- Fluid retention and weight gain: 1 inch superior and lateral to the umbilicus; T12 and L1 lamina
- Anxiety: third, fourth, fifth, and sixth intercostal spaces; T3–7 lamina

Spinal Manipulation

- Manipulative techniques to the upper cervical spine and sacrum to boost parasympathetic activity.
- Techniques such as spinal touch and Logan basic for "sympathetic dominance"–related symptoms.

Hormone Therapy

Progesterone creams to modulate the effects of estrogen dominance. Progesterone creams in nonmenopausal women should be introduced during the luteal phase beginning on or around day 12 and extending through day 26. A low dose (approximately 15 to 20 mg/day) of the cream should be applied to the cheeks, chin, neck, upper chest, and inner thighs.

Technical Note

Research on oral micronized progesterone in doses of 100 to 400 mg daily shows no improvement for symptoms of PMS.

- Talk therapy and reassurance are integral parts of PMS management.

Medications

- For affective symptoms:
  - Alprazolam 0.25 three times daily
  - Prozac/Sarafem 20 mg/day
  - Paxil 20 mg/day
  - Zoloft 50 to 100 mg/day

- Celexa 20 mg/day
- Effexor 37.5 to 75 mg/day
- Lexapro 10 to 20 mg/day
- For edema:
  - Aldactone 100 mg/day during the luteal phase
- For cyclic mastodynia:
  - Daily oral contraceptives
  - Bromocriptine
  - Tamoxifen

33

Reproductive Tract Malignancies

PREINVASIVE VULVAR CANCER

What Is It?

Malignancy of the vulva is a rare form of cancer that primarily affects the labia.

Who Gets It?

The most common form of vulvar cancer, squamous cell carcinoma, occurs in postmenopausal women in their sixties or seventies. The average age at diagnosis is 65; however, diagnosis can occur in women in their eighties or nineties. Melanoma, which is a rare form of invasive vulvar carcinoma, has been reported in women in their forties.

Other forms of vulvar cancers include basal cell carcinoma (1.4%), adenocarcinoma (1.2%), and sarcoma (2%). Basal cell carcinoma and adenocarcinoma affect the elderly age group, whereas melanomas and sarcomas often arise in premenopausal women.

Etiology

The cause of vulvar carcinoma is unknown; however, there is increasing evidence that the herpes simplex virus and the human papillomavirus may be precursors to vulvar cancer.

Signs and Symptoms

- Pruritus around the vulva
- Vulvar pain

- Bleeding, discharge, or the presence of a lump
- Dysuria and dyspareunia may be present
- Affected areas can be thicker and lighter
- Red, pink, or white bumps
- Darkly pigmented growth
- Mass on either side of the opening of the vagina
- Soreness on the vulva
- Growths on the vulva

Diagnosis

- Pelvic examination and Papanicolaou (Pap) smear, followed by incision biopsy
- Pelvic examination may reveal a lesion or lump close to the Bartholin's gland; palpable lymph nodes may be observed in the inguinal and femoral areas
- Complete blood count (CBC), liver function tests, and renal function tests
- Staging to determine treatment includes a chest radiograph, magnetic resonance imaging (MRI), computed tomography (CT) scan, cystoscopy, proctoscopy, and intravenous pyelogram

Management

- Determined by the stage of the disease—vulvar intraepithelial neoplasia (VIN) I II III.
- Simple vulvectomy.
- Radical vulvectomy with inguinal and femoral lymphadenectomy.
- Modified radical vulvectomy, which involves radical excision of unilateral disease while leaving the contralateral vulva intact, is considered if the squamous cell invasion is less than 5 mm and the lesion is less than 2 cm in diameter.
- Sexual rehabilitation of the patient may be augmented by plastic surgery procedures such as vulvar reconstruction with gracilis flaps or coverage of the inguinal region with tensor fascia lata flaps or skin grafts. Emotional support as necessary is offered.
- The survival rate is 75% at 5 years unless metastasis involves more than three inguinal lymph nodes, in which case the 5-year survival rate is approximately 20%.

VAGINAL CANCER

What Is It?

Vaginal cancer is a rare form of cancer that affects the vagina. Approximately 1% to 2% of all gynecologic malignancies arise in the vagina, of which 95% are squamous cell occurring in women ages 55 to 65, and approximately 2% are adenocarcinomas occurring in younger women with an average age of 19 years.

Who Gets It?

- Squamous cell carcinoma occurs primarily in postmenopausal women ages 55 to 70.
- Adenocarcinoma occurs primarily in younger women with previous exposure to diethylstilbestrol (DES).

Etiology

- The cause of squamous cell carcinoma is unknown.
- Adenocarcinoma and clear cell carcinoma have been linked to in utero exposure to DES before the eighteenth week of gestation.

Signs and Symptoms

- Vaginal bleeding occurs in approximately 60% of cases.

Technical Note

Reproductive tract malignancy should be suspected when there is a resumption of bleeding in a postmenopausal woman who has ceased menses for 1 year in the absence of hormone replacement therapy.

- Increased vaginal discharge
- Color and consistency changes in vaginal discharge in approximately 20% of cases; discharge becomes more watery and brown in color and may cause itching
- Pain on urination
- Pressure in the rectum
- Pain with bowel movements
- Vaginal and bladder pain as the disease progresses

Diagnosis

- Four-quadrant Pap smear
- Colposcopy
- Biopsy
- Chest x-rays, CT scan, and MRI are used for metastasis and staging

Management

- Lesions in the lower vagina may be treated with pelvic exenteration and radical vulvectomy.
- To conserve bladder and rectal function, radiation therapy is recommended for smaller lesions (less than 2 cm).
- Larger lesions are treated with a combination of external beam radiation therapy and interstitial or intracavitary brachytherapy.
- Younger women with adenocarcinoma typically have a lesion in the upper half of the vagina and may be treated by radical hysterectomy with upper vaginectomy combined with pelvic lymphadenectomy.

CERVICAL CANCER

What Is It?

Cervical cancer is malignancy of the cervix, the portion of the uterus that is visible at the top of the vaginal vault. Most cervical cancers arise from the squamous cells on the outer surface of the cervix and the transitional zone. A small proportion of cervical cancer is adenocarcinoma, which arises from the glandular, mucus-secreting cells of the endocervix.

Who Gets It?

Cervical cancer typically is diagnosed in women in their forties or fifties; the average age at diagnosis is 48.

Etiology and Risk Factors

Cervical cancer arises from unmanaged cervical dysplasia. Cervical dysplasia is a precancerous condition that is completely treatable. Risk factors for cervical dysplasia and cervical cancer are as follows.

- History of infection with herpes simplex virus (HSV)
- History of infection with human papillomavirus (HPV)
- Early age of sexual activity
- Multiple sexual partners without the use of barrier methods of birth control
- Smoking
- DES exposure
- Oral contraceptive use

Women who use oral contraceptives may have a higher incidence of cervical dysplasia. Whether this is due to the fact that this group of women is more likely to schedule Pap smears consistently or that they are less likely to use a barrier method of birth control remains undetermined.

Clinical Pearl

HPV has been detected in the sperm of men who had no visible symptoms of HPV. Women with recurrent episodes of cervical dysplasia should have their partners evaluated for HPV.

- Decreased immunity such as observed in chronic systemic diseases (diabetes, human immunodeficiency virus [HIV], kidney failure, etc.) may increase risk for cervical dysplasia
- Sexually transmitted diseases such as chlamydia may increase risk for cervical dysplasia

Signs and Symptoms

- Approximately 70% of women with early-stage cancer have no unusual bleeding, and in approximately 60%, the cervix appears normal
- Vaginal bleeding or spotting that occurs between menses, or as a result of activity such as exercise or straining with bowel movements
- Postcoital bleeding
- Vaginal discharge that is watery, blood tinged, or yellow brown in color
- Invasive cervical cancer often appears as an irregular fleshy growth
- As the condition progresses, the patient experiences pain, pelvic pressure, or rectal pressure

Diagnosis

- By one or several screening/diagnostic procedures:
  - The Pap smear (also known as cervical smear) is a sampling of cells from the cervix that aids in the diagnosis of precancerous cells.
  - The thin prep Pap is similar to the conventional Pap smear in that a sampling of the cells from the cervix is obtained. The sample is deposited into a fluid medium instead of onto a slide, a process that allows for subsequent evaluation for HPV, DNA testing, and simultaneous screening for chlamydia and gonorrhea.
  - Colposcopy involves bathing the cervix in a vinegar water solution and subsequent evaluation under magnification with the use of a colposcope. Colposcopy with biopsy is done to confirm the diagnosis.

Management

Management is determined by the stage of the disease–Cervical Intraepithelial Neoplasia (CIN) I II III.

Screening

Screening–regular Pap smears (see following guidelines).

- Stress management. Mild cervical dysplasia may be an indication of excessive stress.
- Diet and nutritional supplementation to enhance overall immune health should be recommended.
- Folate supplementation. In a clinical trial, folic acid supplementation of 10 mg per day resulted in improvement or normalization of Pap smears in women with cervical dysplasia. The rate of normalization for women with untreated cervical dysplasia is typically 1.3% for mild dysplasia and 0% for moderate dysplasia. In clinical trials, treatment with folic acid showed the regression to normal rate at 20% in one study and 100% in another. The progression rate of cervical dysplasia in untreated patients is approximately 16% at 4 months. In the folate-supplemented group, none of the participants progressed. Folate supplementation for mild dysplasia in the absence of clear evidence of HPV might be useful. The recommended dose is 10 mg of folic acid daily.

Treatment

Medical management is dependent on the severity of the cervical cancer.

- Treatments for noninvasive cancers include the following:
  - Cone biopsy.
  - Cryotherapy.
  - In the loop electrosurgical excision procedure (LEEP), also known as large loop excision of the cervix (LLEC) and loop cone biopsy, a special wire loop connected to an electrical source is used to evaluate and remove predetermined areas of abnormality on the cervix. The procedure requires local anesthesia.
- Treatments for invasive cancers include the following:
  - Microinvasive carcinoma. The lesion typically is less than 3 mm, and the probability of lymphatic metastasis is less than 1%. Treatment is by extrafascial vaginal or abdominal hysterectomy.
  - Invasive carcinoma. Procedures used depend on the severity of the condition, the age of the patient, the ability of the patient to tolerate radical surgery, and additional factors such as the desire to preserve ovarian function, vaginal function, and sexual satisfaction.
  - Radiation therapy involves high doses of radiation to the pelvis in the form of external beam irradiation and intracavitary irradiation (brachytherapy). Generally the pelvic viscera can tolerate relatively high doses of radiation before complications arise. *Brachytherapy* means "short therapy" and involves implanting radioactive sources in or near the malignancy. Brachytherapy is available in both high dose rate (HDR) and low dose rate (LDR).
  - Radical hysterectomy (Wertheim hysterectomy) involves complete resection of the uterus, cervix, and parametrial tissues.
  - Pelvic lymphadenectomy is performed for both staging and treatment purposes, and involves extensive dissection of the base of the bladder and terminal ureter, as well as deep pelvic dissection. Hemorrhage and injury to the bladder, ureter, or rectum are potential complications.

Prevention

- Early diagnosis of cervical dysplasia
- Regular Pap smears
- Use of barrier methods of birth control such as condoms, diaphragms, and cervical caps
- Avoid intercourse if visible warts are apparent on the partner's genitals

Pap smear guidelines. American Cancer Society guidelines for Pap smear are as follows:

- Women who have been sexually active and have a cervix should be regularly screened.
- All asymptomatic women age 20 and over, and those under 20 who are sexually active, should have a Pap test annually for two negative examinations and then at least every 3 years until age 65.
- A pelvic examination should be done as part of a general physical examination every 3 years from age 20 to 40 and annually thereafter.
- Women at high risk for developing endometrial cancer should have a Pap test at menopause.

The August 2005 American College of Obstetricians and Gynecologists (ACOG) guidelines are as follows:

- First Pap smear: approximately three years after first sexual encounter, or by age 21, whichever comes first.
- Women up to age 30: annual Pap smear. Because this group has the greatest risk of HPV, yearly testing still is recommended.
- Women over age 30: a negative Pap smear for 3 consecutive years means future testing is necessary only every 2 to 3 years.
- One negative test result using a combined Pap smear and specific HPV test means future screening is necessary every 3 years thereafter. If one of the two tests is positive, more frequent screening may be necessary.
- Exceptions: Women who are HIV positive, were exposed to DES in utero, or have suppressed immune systems still need yearly testing.
- Women with a hysterectomy: if the cervix is removed, and there is no evidence of malignancy and no history of abnormal cancerous cell growth, Pap smears can be discontinued.
- If there is a previous history of abnormal cervical cell growth, annual screening is recommended until there are three consecutive negative tests, after which screening can be discontinued.

The new guidelines also stress more individualized treatment of women, with physicians determining on a case-by-case basis who can stop having cervical cancer screenings, and at what age. Important factors to consider include the woman's age, her medical history, and her health care status.

OVARIAN CANCER

What Is It?

Ovarian cancer is an umbrella term for several different malignancies of the ovaries. Each of these cancers has different characteristics, treatments, and survival rates. Epithelial ovarian cancer arises from the germinal epithelium of the ovary, makes up approximately 80% of ovarian cancers, and occurs primarily in postmenopausal women, but it can occur as early as the midthirties.

Who Gets It?

The other forms of ovarian cancer are germ cell cancers, which occur primarily during childhood and adolescence, and gonadal, mesenchymal, stromal, and sex cord tumors, which are much less common and can arise anytime throughout the woman's lifetime (although more commonly in women over age 35). One quarter of all ovarian cancer deaths occur in women ages 35 to 54, and half of all ovarian cancer deaths occur in women ages 55 to 75.

Etiology

- The cause of ovarian cancer is unknown; however, it appears that women with the breast cancer genes BRCA1 or BRCA2 or with a history of breast cancer are at higher risk.
- There is controversial evidence to suggest that the use of talcum powder, living in industrialized nations, and the use of fertility drugs might increase the risk for ovarian cancer.
- Epithelial ovarian cancer is thought to be linked to ovulation. This hypothesis appears to be supported by the increased risk of developing epithelial ovarian cancer that is observed in nulliparous women and diminished risk in women who have had two or more pregnancies.

Clinical Pearl

Pregnancy, lactation, use of oral contraceptives, and other scenarios in which the ovaries gain physiologic rest appear to decrease the risk for ovarian cancer.

Signs and Symptoms

Signs and symptoms, when they occur, include the following:

- Abdominal pain
- Abdominal swelling
- Irregularities in bladder and bowel function
- Varicose veins
- Hemorrhoids
- Swelling of the legs or vulva
- Feelings of fullness or heaviness in the pelvic region
- Changes in weight
- Low back pain
- Vaginal bleeding
- Serosanguineous vaginal discharge
- Gastrointestinal symptoms such as flatulence, indigestion, loss of appetite, nausea, and vomiting

Many of the symptoms of ovarian cancer appear to be related to the gastrointestinal tract. This is due in part to the fact that ovarian cancers shed malignant cells, which then implant on organs of the reproductive and gastrointestinal systems, including the uterus, bladder, bowels, and omentum. These cells become sites for additional tumor growth.

Diagnosis

- Screening by way of regular pelvic examinations.
- Pelvic ultrasound.
- Blood tests for the ovarian cancer–associated antigen, CA 125. A palpable adnexal mass on pelvic examination with an elevated CA 125 is positive for ovarian cancer in 80% of patients.
- Definitive diagnosis of ovarian cancer is based on surgical exploration by laparotomy and pathologic review.
- Diagnosis by symptomatology is difficult because symptoms are vague and often mimic gastrointestinal disorders. As a result, by the time the woman seeks treatment, the disease

often has progressed to other areas of the reproductive tract and abdominal cavity.
- Additional diagnostic protocols might include CBC, human chorionic gonadotropin (HCG), alpha-fetoprotein, urinalysis, a complete gastrointestinal series, abdominal CT or MRI scan, and ultrasound.

Management

Prevention strategies include the following:
- Dietary folate. Results of a study conducted in Sweden indicate that high levels of folate obtained from food sources may protect against ovarian cancer. In this study of more than 60,000 women, 266 of whom developed ovarian cancer, women with the highest levels of folate in their diet (at least 204 mcg/day) were 33% less likely to develop ovarian cancer than those with the lowest levels (less than 155 mcg/day). Among women who consumed more than two drinks per week, the risk reduction seen with folate intake was 74%.
- Acetaminophen. There is some evidence that the pain killer acetaminophen may lower ovarian cancer risk. In a study of women who regularly used acetaminophen, there was a 50% to 60% decrease in ovarian cancer when compared with those who did not.

Medical management. Treatment depends on a number of factors, such as stage and grade of the disease, the patient's age, and the patient's overall health.

Treatment typically involves surgical removal of the ovaries followed by chemotherapy or radiation (or both). The chemotherapeutic regimens are intense and patients often encounter severe toxicity. Complications include pancytopenia, sepsis, alopecia, hepatic toxicity, pulmonary toxicity, neurotoxicity, nephrotoxicity, and, in the long term, pulmonary fibrosis and even leukemia.

Survival rate for ovarian cancer is poor (approximately 15% at 5 years) because of the spread via epithelium and lymphatic channels into the peritoneal/abdominal cavity as a result of delayed diagnosis. If diagnosis is made while the malignancy remains confined to the ovaries, survival rate is approximately 90%.

FALLOPIAN TUBE CANCER

What Is It?

Malignancy of the fallopian tube is the rarest of all the gynecologic malignancies, accounting for 0.1% to 0.5% of the gynecologic cancers.

Who Gets It?

Typically women of low parity with an average age at diagnosis of 55 years.

Signs and Symptoms

Signs and symptoms, although vague, may elicit a history of mild but chronic lower abdominal and pelvic pain, vaginal bleeding, and vaginal discharge.

Diagnosis

Physical examination may reveal an adnexal mass. Because fallopian tube cancer is so rare, it may be suspected in a patient with Pap smear evidence of adenocarcinoma and negative fractional dilation and curettage (D&C).

Treatment

Treatment for fallopian tube cancer is similar to that outlined for epithelial ovarian cancer and may involve total abdominal hysterectomy, bilateral salpingo-oophorectomy, omentectomy, peritoneal cytology, and selective lymphadenectomy followed by chemotherapeutic agents.

The overall survival rate is approximately 18% for stage III disease and between 40% and 75% for stage I and II disease.

UTERINE CANCER

What Is It?

Also known as endometrial cancer, uterine cancers are malignancies primarily of the endometrial lining of the uterus. Uterine cancer is the leading invasive gynecologic malignancy encountered in the United States. Approximately 38,000 cases are diagnosed yearly.

Who Gets It?

Most uterine cancers (approximately 75%) occur in postmenopausal women. Less than 3% occur in women 40 years of age and younger.

Etiology

The primary cause of endometrial cancer appears to be unopposed or excess estrogen. Risk factors include the following:
- Obesity
- Late menopause (after age 53)
- Nulliparity
- Hypertension
- Diabetes
- Ovarian disorders such as polycystic ovary syndrome and granulosa tumors of the ovary
- Previous history of reproductive and other cancers
- Hereditary
- Early menarche or late menopause (or both)
- History of benign polyps or other growths of the endometrial lining
- High-fat diet
- Estrogen replacement therapy (ERT)

   Case-controlled studies in the early 1970s revealed that the risk of developing endometrial carcinoma in patients taking ERT was increased from threefold to twelvefold. This risk is tied closely to the dosage and duration of ERT.

   There is some evidence that tamoxifen (given to treat breast cancer) may increase the risk of uterine cancer.

Signs and Symptoms

The most common symptom of uterine cancer is abnormal bleeding. Painless vaginal bleeding is a hallmark of uterine cancer and occurs in 90% of cases. Uterine cancer should be considered in any case of a postmenopausal woman who has stopped bleeding for more than 1 year, and resumes bleeding in the absence of hormone replacement therapy. Bleeding between periods in premenopausal women also may be an indication.

Additional symptoms include pelvic pain, lower abdominal pain, low-grade and diffuse low back pain, pelvic mass, serosanguineous vaginal discharge, and vaginal discharge that may be profuse and malodorous and may occur in bursts, particularly after heavy exertion or straining.

Diagnosis

Diagnosis of uterine cancer is based on the following:
- Symptoms of vaginal bleeding
- Pap smear
- Endometrial and endocervical biopsy
- Fractional D&C performed under general or spinal anesthesia

Management

Before initiating treatment for uterine cancer, it is important to evaluate disease progression. Staging is as follows:

Stage 1. Cancer is confined to the uterus.

Stage 2. Cancer is limited to the uterus and cervix.

Stage 3. Cancer extends outside the uterus to the reproductive organs and may involve lymph nodes in the pelvis and abdominal aorta.

Stage 4. Cancer has spread to the inner surface of the bowel, bladder, abdomen, and other distant organs.

Women with stage 1 disease typically are treated with abdominal hysterectomy, including bilateral salpingo-oophorectomy. This is performed to accommodate the spread of the malignant cells to the ovaries and to avoid stimulation of dormant cancer cells by estrogen production from the ovaries. Abdominal hysterectomy is the preferred choice of surgery because it affords the opportunity to examine and obtain washings of the abdominal cavity to detect any further evidence of cancer.

Women with stage 2 disease and those with stage 1 disease who are at increased risk for recurrence are treated with surgery and combination radiation therapy.

Treatment for women with stage 3 and 4 disease typically involves surgery, radiation therapy, and possibly chemotherapy or hormonal therapy such as progestins or antiestrogens.

The 5-year survival rates are as follows:

Stage	Percent of Total Cases	5-Year Survival
1	74%	>72% (75%–90%)
2	14%	56%
3	6%	31%
4	3%	<9%

Treatment of recurrent disease involves the antiestrogen drug tamoxifen or progestin therapy. Hormonal therapies usually are the first choice for treating distant metastases. Chemotherapy is an added option.

34

Vulvodynia

WHAT IS IT?

Vulvodynia is an all-encompassing term to describe several conditions, including cyclic vulvovaginitis, vulvar vestibulitis syndrome, and essential vulvodynia, all of which manifest with acute or chronic vulvar pain.

WHO GETS IT?

Vulvodynia appears to afflict primarily Caucasian women.

ETIOLOGY

Unknown. Proposed causes include the following:
- Allergic reactions to food, feminine hygiene products, soaps, toilet paper, other sanitary products, and clothing fibers
- Previous vaginal infections
- Irritation or injury to the nerves around the vulva
- Autoimmune disorders
- Chronic tension
- Muscle spasms
- Sexual abuse
- History of cryotherapy to the vulva
- History of laser therapy to the vulva
- Lichen sclerosis

Technical Note

Lichen sclerosis is a condition that causes inflammation and white plaques on the vulva and progressive pruritus, dyspareunia, dysuria, or genital bleeding. The inflammation can be so intense that it causes blisters, which may mimic the trauma of sexual abuse or other genital ulcerative disease. Autoimmune causes are suspected to be the primary cause of lichen sclerosis.

SIGNS AND SYMPTOMS

- Raw feeling around the vulva
- Vulvar burning, soreness, itching, or stinging
- Dyspareunia
- The pain in the vulva frequently is aggravated by activities of daily living

DIAGNOSIS

- Detailed history
- Physical examination, including pelvic examination
- Screening for bacterial, viral, and fungal infections

MANAGEMENT

Lifestyle Factors

- Avoid potential allergens such as soaps, vaginal creams, and feminine deodorant sprays
- Wear cotton underwear
- Wear loose clothing
- Frequent washing of the genital area with water alone
- Avoid deodorized sanitary products
- Avoid tight-fitting clothing, including underwear, panty hose, and jeans
- Apply cold compresses directly to the genital area
- Take sitz baths
- Avoid exercises that put direct pressure on the vulva, such as bicycling
- Follow a low-oxalate diet
- Take supplementary calcium citrate

Therapy

- Physical therapy, including biofeedback and other relaxation training procedures, to release pelvic muscles in spasm and to decrease the pain response
- Pelvic strengthening exercises and therapies
- Spinal manipulation as needed to release irritation to the spinal nerves supplying the vulva

MEDICATIONS

- Local anesthetics for pain relief
- Cortisone and other topical creams
- Antihistamines to reduce itching
- Antidepressants for chronic pain
- Estrogen creams
- Treatment for identified infections or fungi

SUPPORT

- Vulvar pain support groups

Appendix

IN UTERO CONSTRAINT (WEBSTER TECHNIQUE)

The patient lies prone on the examining table. The health care provider flexes both of the patient's knees to bring the heels to the buttocks. If both knees are symmetric, the procedure is discontinued. If one side is restricted, the sacrum on the restricted side is adjusted for posterior rotation. The patient then is instructed to lie supine. The provider evaluates for a trigger point–like nodule in the round ligament on the side of posterior rotation of the sacrum. To locate this point, an imaginary diagonal line is drawn from the anterior superior iliac spine (ASIS) toward the symphysis pubis and from the navel toward the anterior inferior iliac spine (AIIS). The point of intersection of these two lines is the approximate location of this nodule. The nodule is massaged until it releases. No further treatment is given. The patient may need to have the procedure repeated on subsequent visits.

The Webster technique should be performed by a health care provider certified in the technique. For information on certification, see the website www.icpa4kids.com.

PELVIC FLOOR (KEGEL EXERCISES)

To identify the correct muscles, the patient places a clean finger in the vagina, squeezes the finger, and identifies the muscles that contract around the finger. Next, the patient attempts to stop the flow of urine using just the pelvic floor muscles while urinating and identifies the muscles used for this maneuver. These are the core muscle groups used in the pelvic floor exercises.

Once the muscles have been identified, the exercises are performed a minimum of three times daily. The patient contracts the muscles and sustains the contraction for 10 seconds followed by 10 seconds of rest. The cycle is repeated 10 times.

Additional guidelines:

- The exercise is best performed seated or standing, not supine.
- The exercise should be performed with an empty bladder.

- It is important to use only the pelvic floor muscles and to avoid recruiting the quadriceps, gluteus muscles, and abdominals.
- The exercise should not cause strain. The patient should be relaxed during the exercise and breathe freely.
- Once the muscles have been identified, the exercise should not be performed while urinating because this can result in weaker muscles, incomplete emptying of the bladder, and bladder infections.
- Vaginal cones may be used to enhance the exercise.

BUCKLED SACRUM MANEUVER*

The buckled sacrum maneuver, as described by Dr. C.J. Phillips for relief of symptoms associated with increased pressure on the cervix, is as follows:

The mother stands several feet from a wall, facing the wall. Her feet are shoulder width apart. She rests her hands against the wall.

The helper stands perpendicular to the mother with one hand just above the pubic region and the other hand on the lumbosacral spine, fingers pointed toward the floor. The hand on the back applies slight pressure and slides down the lumbosacral and sacroiliac area. If the palm of the hand feels any resistance to the downward motion, downward pressure against the sacrum is maintained for several minutes or until the buckled sacral segments smooth out and the hand slides down without resistance. The hormones of pregnancy, combined with pressure against the segments, allow the pliable sacrum to mold to the contour of the hand. This is an extremely gentle maneuver. No pressure is applied toward the baby by either hand.

When the sacral segments realign, balance is restored to the uterine ligaments and the uterus no longer applies pressure against the structures located in the front of the abdomen, resulting in resolution of the premature contractions and thigh pain.

Some patients are able to correct the buckled sacrum themselves by lying on the floor with a small rolled towel about

---

*Copyright: Phillips CJ: *Hands of Love, Seven Steps to the Miracle of Birth* 1st ed, St. Paul, 2001, New Dawn Publishing.

2 inches high and 4 inches wide slipped under their lower back. They slide the towel downward until the buckled segment of the sacrum restricts it; the weight of the mother's body resting on the towel works to help the sacrum realign itself.

Four Steps to Reduce Back Labor*

1. The mother lies on her side at the edge of a table with the bottom leg straight and the head resting on a pillow. The examiner stands with his or her legs straddling the mother's belly.
2. The mother's hips and shoulders should be straight and perfectly perpendicular to the spine.
3. The mother drops the top leg off the table and allows it to hang downward for a few minutes. The provider hooks his or her thumbs into the anterior superior iliac spine (ASIS) while applying downward pressure to the ilia.

   The resultant separation of the sacroiliac (SI) joint frees the sacrum and decreases the tone of the pelvic floor muscles, which may free the baby's head, allowing it to turn from the pubic bone.
4. After a few minutes, the mother rolls over to her other side and the procedure is repeated.

   At home, the mother may be able to kneel on a step with her forearms on the floor and the hips above the head. The water floats toward the lungs, and the baby's head dislodges enough from the pelvic outlet to be able to rotate the face away from the pubic bone.

   This technique does not work if
   - The cord is wrapped tightly around the body, thereby restricting movements
   - The extremities are trapped in a distorted position
   - The infant is induced before the cranium has molded

SACRAL NERVE STIMULATION

This technique is a surgical procedure used to treat incontinence that is not responsive to other treatments. Specifically used to treat urge incontinence and urinary frequency, sacral nerve stim-

---

*Copyright: Phillips CJ: *Hands of Love, Seven Steps to the Miracle of Birth* 1st ed, St. Paul, 2001, New Dawn Publishing.

ulation generally is not recommended for people with stress incontinence or men with overflow incontinence. A small electrical device is used to transmit electrical impulses to the sacral nerve in order to decrease urgency. The system is surgically placed under the skin once efficacy has been established.

Table 8-1/11-1

Body Mass Index

BMI	Normal						Overweight					Obese						
	19	20	21	22	23	24	25	26	27	28	29	30	31	32	33	34	35	36
Height (inches)									Body Weight (pounds)									
58	91	96	100	105	110	115	119	124	129	134	138	143	148	153	158	162	167	172
59	94	99	104	109	114	119	124	128	133	138	143	148	153	158	163	168	173	178
60	97	102	107	112	118	123	128	133	138	143	148	153	158	163	168	174	179	184
61	100	106	111	116	122	127	132	137	143	148	153	158	164	169	174	180	185	190
62	104	109	115	120	126	131	136	142	147	153	158	164	169	175	180	186	191	196
63	107	113	118	124	130	135	141	146	152	158	163	169	175	180	186	191	197	203
64	110	116	122	128	134	140	145	151	157	163	169	174	180	186	192	197	204	209
65	114	120	126	132	138	144	150	156	162	168	174	180	186	192	198	204	210	216
66	118	124	130	136	142	148	155	161	167	173	179	186	192	198	204	210	216	223
67	121	127	134	140	146	153	159	166	172	178	185	191	198	204	211	217	223	230
68	125	131	138	144	151	158	164	171	177	184	190	197	203	210	216	223	230	236
69	128	135	142	149	155	162	169	176	182	189	196	203	209	216	223	230	236	243
70	132	139	146	153	160	167	174	181	188	195	202	209	216	222	229	236	243	250
71	136	143	150	157	165	172	179	186	193	200	208	215	222	229	236	243	250	257
72	140	147	154	162	169	177	184	191	199	206	213	221	228	235	242	250	258	265
73	144	151	159	166	174	182	189	197	204	212	219	227	235	242	250	257	265	272
74	148	155	163	171	179	186	194	202	210	218	225	233	241	249	256	264	272	280
75	152	160	168	176	184	192	200	208	216	224	232	240	248	256	264	272	279	287
76	156	164	172	180	189	197	205	213	221	230	238	246	254	263	272	279	287	295
58	177	181	186	191	196	201	205	210	215	220	224	229	234	239	244	248	253	258

(continued)

Table 8-1/11-1

Body Mass Index—cont'd

BMI	Normal						Overweight					Obese						
	19	20	21	22	23	24	25	26	27	28	29	30	31	32	33	34	35	36
Height (inches)							Body Weight (pounds)											
59	183	188	193	198	203	208	212	217	222	227	232	237	242	247	252	257	262	267
60	189	194	199	204	209	215	220	225	230	235	240	245	250	255	261	266	271	276
61	195	201	206	211	217	222	227	232	238	243	248	254	259	264	269	275	280	285
62	202	207	213	218	224	229	235	240	246	251	256	262	267	273	278	284	289	295
63	208	214	220	225	231	237	242	248	254	259	265	270	276	282	287	293	299	304
64	215	221	227	232	238	244	250	256	262	267	273	279	285	291	296	302	308	314
65	222	228	234	240	246	252	258	264	270	276	282	288	294	300	306	312	318	324
66	229	235	241	247	253	260	266	272	278	284	291	297	303	309	315	322	328	334
67	236	242	249	255	261	268	274	280	287	293	299	306	312	319	325	331	338	344
68	243	249	256	262	269	276	282	289	295	302	308	315	322	328	335	341	348	354
69	250	257	263	270	277	284	291	297	304	311	318	324	331	338	345	351	358	365
70	257	264	271	278	285	292	299	306	313	320	327	334	341	348	355	362	369	376
71	265	272	279	286	293	301	308	315	322	329	338	343	351	358	365	372	379	386
72	272	279	287	294	302	309	316	324	331	338	346	353	361	368	375	383	390	397
73	280	288	295	302	310	318	325	333	340	348	355	363	371	378	386	393	401	408
74	287	295	303	311	319	326	334	342	350	358	365	373	381	389	396	404	412	420
75	295	303	311	319	327	335	343	351	359	367	375	383	391	399	407	415	423	431
76	304	312	320	328	336	344	353	361	369	377	385	394	402	410	418	426	435	443

From *Clinical guidelines on the identification, evaluation, and treatment of overweight and obesity in adults: evidence report*, NIH pub no 98-4083. Published by the National Heart, Lung, and Blood Institute (NHLBI) and available through the NHLBI Health Information Center, PO Box 30105, Bethesda, MD 20824-0105; 301-592-8573; www.nhlbi.nih.gov.

Bibliography

ANATOMY, PHYSIOLOGY, AND NEUROLOGY

Chappell PE, White RS, Mellon PL: Circadian gene expression regulates pulsatile gonadotrophin releasing hormone secretory patterns in the hypothalamic GNRH secreting Gt1-7 cell line, *J Neurosci* 23(35):11202–11213, 2003.

Clarke-Pearson DL, Dawood MY: *Green's gynecology: essentials of clinical practice*, ed 4, Boston, 1990, Little, Brown.

Gray H: *Gray's anatomy*, Philadelphia, 1973 Lea & Febiger.

Marshall JC et al: Gonadotropin-releasing hormone pulses: regulators of gonadotropin synthesis and ovulatory cycles, *Recent Prog Horm Res* 47:155–189, 1991.

Scott JR, Gibbs RS, Karlan BY, Haney AF: *Danforth's obstetrics and gynecology*, ed 9, Philadelphia, 2003, Lippincott Williams & Wilkins.

Shephard BD, Shephard CA: *The complete guide to women's health*, ed 2 , New York, 1990, Plume.

Speroff L, Fritz MA: *Clinical gynecologic endocrinology and infertility*, ed 7, Philadelphia, 2005, Lippincott Williams & Wilkins.

Youngkin EQ, Davis MS: *Women's health: a primary care clinical guide*, ed 2, Stamford, CT, 1998, Appleton & Lange.

ESTROGEN CONCEPTS

Alanko J et al: Catechol estrogens as inhibitors of leukotriene synthesis, *Biochem Pharmacol* 55(1):101–104, 1998.

Bradlow HL: 2-hydroxyestrone: the good estrogen, *J Endocrinol* 150(suppl): S259–S265, 1996.

Colborn T, Dumanoski D, Myers JP: *Our stolen future*, New York, 1996, Penguin.

Kall MA et al: Effects of dietary broccoli on human in vivo drug metabolizing enzymes: evaluation of caffeine, oestrone and chlorzoxazone metabolism, *Carcinogenesis* 17(4):793–799, 1996.

Moggs JG et al: The need to decide if all estrogens are intrinsically similar, *Environ Health Perspect* 112(11):1137–1142, 2004.

MENSTRUAL CYCLE

Baerwald AR, Adams GP, Pierson RA: A new model for ovarian follicular development during the human menstrual cycle, *Fertil Steril* 80:1, 2003.

Besser GM, Mortimer CH: Hypothalamic regulatory hormones: a review, *J Clin Pathol* 27(3):173–184, 1974.

Bjerke CA, Goldschmidt SB: *The collection of writings by J. Lamoine DeRusha*, ed 1, Bloomington, 1984, NWCC Alumni Association.

Clarke-Pearson DL, Dawood MY: *Green's gynecology: essentials of clinical practice*, ed 4, Boston, 1990, Little, Brown.

Dunson DB, Colombo B, Baird DD: Changes with age in the level and duration of fertility in the menstrual cycle, *J Human Reproduction* 17(5):1399–1403, 2002.

Emans JS, Laufer M, Goldstein DP: Delayed puberty and menstrual irregularities, *Pediatric and Adolescent Gynecology*, ed 4, Philadelphia, 1998, Lippincott-Raven.

Filicori M, Butler JP, Crowley WR Jr: Neuroendocrine regulation of the corpus luteum in the human. Evidence for pulsatile progesterone secretion, *J Clin Invest* 73(6):1638-1647, 1984.

Gomel V, Munro MG, Rowe T: *Gynecology: a practical approach*, Baltimore, 1990, Williams & Wilkins.

Harlow SD, Campbell OM: Epidemiology of menstrual disorders in developing countries: a systematic review, *BJOG* 111(1):6-16, 2004.

Herman-Giddens M et al: Secondary sexual characteristics and menses in young girls seen in office practice, *Pediatrics,* April 1997, p 505.

Hotchkiss J, Knobil E: The menstrual cycle and its neuroendocrine control. In Knobil E, Neill JD, editors: *The physiology of reproduction*, ed 2, New York, 1994, Raven.

Lemcke DP et al: *Primary care of women*, Norwalk, CT, 1995, Appleton & Lange.

Ling FW, Duff P: *Obstetrics and gynecology principles for practice*, New York, 2001, McGraw-Hill.

Marti O, Armario A: Anterior pituitary response to stress: time-related changes and adaptation, *Int J Dev Neurosci* 16(3-4):241-260, 1998.

Ouyang F et al: Serum DDT, age at menarche, and abnormal menstrual cycle length, *Occup Environ Med* 62:878-884, 2005.

Reis E, Frick U, Schmidtbleicher D: Frequency variations of strength training session triggered by the phases of the menstrual cycle, *Int J Sports Med* 16: 545-550, 1995.

Rossmanith WG, Gambacciani M: Autonomous gonadotrophin release from the human pituitary in vitro and factors influencing this secretion, *Gynecol Endocrinol* 8(4):265-275i, 1994.

Shephard BD, Shephard CA: *The complete guide to women's health*, ed 2, New York, 1990, Plume.

Sherman BM, Korenman SG: Hormonal characteristics of the human menstrual cycle throughout reproductive life, *J Clin Invest* 55(4):699-706, 1975.

Smith MA, Shimp LA: *20 common problems in women's health care*, New York, 2000, McGraw-Hill.

Treloar AE, Boynton RE, Behn DG, Brown BW: Variations of the human menstrual cycle through reproductive life, *Int J Fertil* 12(1 pt 2):77-126, 1967.

Vollman RF: The menstrual cycle. In *Major problems of obstetrics and gynecology*, Philadelphia, 1977, WB Saunders.

Wang RY, Needham LL, Barr DB: Effects of environmental agents on the attainment of puberty: considerations when assessing exposure to environmental chemicals in the National Children's Study, *Environ Health Perspect* 113 (8):1100-1107, 2005.

Wilcox AJ, Dunson D, Baird DD: The timing of the "fertile window" in the menstrual cycle: day specific estimates from a prospective study, *BMJ* 321:1259-1262, 2000.

Women's curse: a general internist's approach to common menstrual problems, *West J Med* 138(1):76-82, 1983.

AMENORRHEA

Aloi JA: Evaluation of amenorrhea, *Compr Ther* 21(10):575, 1995.

Amann W: Amenorrhea. Favorable effect of *agnus castus* on amenorrhea, *ZFA* (Stuttgart) 58(4):228-231, 1982.

Brown RP, Gerbarg PL, Ramazanov DS: Rhodiola rosea: a phytomedicinal overview, *Herbalgram J Am Botan Council* 56:40-52, 2002.

Federman DD: Symposium on adolescent gynecology and endocrinology. Part I. Physiology of sexual maturation and primary amenorrhea, *West J Med* 131 (5):411–416, 1979.
Hudson T: Menstrual disorders. Presented at the Institute of Women's Health and Integrative Medicine, Portland, OR, October 21–23, 2005.
Martin MC, Schriock ED, Jaffe RB: Prolactin-secreting pituitary adenomas, *West J Med* 139(5):663–672, 1983.
Milewicz A et al: *Vitex agnus castus* extract in the treatment of luteal phase defects due to latent hyperprolactinemia. Results of a randomized placebo-controlled double-blind study, *Arzneim Forsch/Drug Res* 43(7):752–756, 1993.
Neinstein LS: Menstrual dysfunction in pathophysiologic states, *West J Med* 143 (4):476–484, 1985.
Sliutz G, Speiser P, Schultz AM, Spona J, Zellinger R: Agnus castus extracts inhibit prolactin secretion of rat pituitary cells, *J Horm Metab Res* 25:253–255, 1993.
Sliutz G, Speiser P, Schultz AM, Spona J, Zellinger RF et al: Serum DDT, age at menarche, and abnormal menstrual cycle length, *Occup Environ Med* 62:878–884, 2005.
Speroff L, Fritz MA: *Clinical gynecologic endocrinology and infertility*, ed 7, Philadelphia, 2005, Lippincott Williams & Wilkins.
Zavanelli-Morgan BA: Amenorrhea. Presentation at Institute of Women's Health and Integrative Medicine, Portland, OR, October 2005.

BIRTH CONTROL

Baird DT, Glasier AF: Contraception, *BMJ* 319(7215):969–972, 1999.
Baird DT, Glasier AF: The science, medicine, and future of contraception, *West J Med* 172(5):321–324, 2000.
Charlafti I: A right for family planning: the benefits of contraception for women's health and social status, *EMBO Rep* 3(3):211–213, 2002.
Gaillard RC, Riondel A, Muller AF, Herrmann W, Baulieu EE: RU 486: a steroid with anti-glucocorticosteroid activity that only disinhibits the human pituitary-adrenal system at a specific time of day, *Proc Natl Acad Sci USA* 81(12):3879–3882, 1984.
Hinks LJ, Clayton BE, Lloyd RS: Zinc and copper concentrations in leucocytes and erythrocytes in healthy adults and the effect of oral contraceptives, *J Clin Pathol* 36(9):1016–1021, 1983.
McGregor JA, Hammill HA: Contraceptive choices for women with medical problems: contraception and sexually transmitted disease: interactions and opportunities, *Am J Obstet Gynecol* 168(suppl):2033, 1993.
Planned Parenthood: www.plannedparenthood.com.
Prasad AS, Lei KY, Moghissi KS, Stryker JC, Oberleas D: Effect of oral contraceptives on nutrients. III. Vitamins B_6, B_{12}, and folic acid, *Am J Obstet Gynecol* 125(8):1063–1069, 1976.
Talwar GP et al: A vaccine that prevents pregnancy in women, *Proc Natl Acad Sci USA* 91(18):8532–8536, 1994.

BLADDER PAIN SYNDROME (INTERSTITIAL CYSTITIS)

Al Hadithi HN et al: Absence of bacterial and viral DNA in bladder biopsies from patients with interstitial cystitis/chronic pelvic pain syndrome, *J Urol* 174(1): 151–154, 2005.

Chuang YC et al: Botulinum toxin treatment of urethral and bladder dysfunction, *J Formos Med Assoc* 102(1):5–11, 2003.

Kusek JW, Nyberg LM: The epidemiology of interstitial cystitis: is it time to expand our definition? *Urology* 57(6 suppl 1):95–99, 2001.

Lorenzo Gomez MF, Gomez Castro S: Physiopathologic relationship between interstitial cystitis and rheumatic, autoimmune, and chronic inflammatory diseases, *Arch Esp Urol* 57(1):25–34, 2004.

Parsons JK, Parsons CL: The historical origins of interstitial cystitis, *J Urol* 171(1): 20–22, 2004.

Shulman L: Female interstitial cystitis: chronic pelvic pain, diagnosis and misdiagnosis, *OB/GYN and Women's Health* 4(5), 2006.

BREAST CONDITIONS

Adebamowo CA et al: Waist-hip ratio and breast cancer risk in urbanized Nigerian women, *Breast Cancer Res* 5(2):R18–R24, 2003.

Baer HJ et al: Body fatness during childhood and adolescence and incidence of breast cancer in premenopausal women: a prospective cohort study, *Breast Cancer Res* 7(3):R314–R325, 2005.

Blommers J, de Lange–De Klerk ES, Kuik DJ et al: Evening primrose oil and fish oil for severe chronic mastalgia: a randomized, double-blind, controlled trial, *Am J Obstet Gynecol* 187(5):1389–1394, 2002.

Bohlke K, Spiegelman D, Trichopoulou A, Katsouyanni K, Trichopoulos D: Vitamins A, C and E and the risk of breast cancer: results from a case-control study in Greece, *Br J Cancer* 79(1):23–29, 1999.

Boyd NP et al: Effects at two years of a low fat, high carbohydrate diet on radiologic features of the breast: results from a randomized trial, *J Natl Cancer Inst* 89(7):488–496, 1997.

Burdina LM: Benign breast diseases: diagnosis and treatment, *Ter Arkh* 70(10): 37–41, 1998.

Dixon-Shanies D, Shaikh N: Growth inhibition of human breast cancer cells by herbs and phytoestrogens, *Oncol Rep* 6(6):1383–1387, 1999.

Feigelson HS, Henderson BE: Future possibilities in the prevention of breast cancer: role of genetic variation in breast cancer prevention, *Breast Cancer Res* 2(4):277–282, 2000.

Gateley CA, Pye JK, Harrison BJ et al: Evening primrose oil (Efamol), a safe treatment option for breast disease, *Breast Cancer Res Treat* 14:161, 2001.

Ghent WR et al: Iodine replacement in fibrocystic disease of the breast, *Can J Surg* 36(5):453–460, 1993.

Greenwald P et al: Fat caloric intake and obesity: lifestyle risk factors and breast cancer, *J Am Diet Assoc* 97:24–30, 1997.

Halaska M, Beles P, Gorkow C et al: Treatment of cyclical mastalgia with a solution containing a *Vitex agnus castus* extract: results of a placebo-controlled double-blind study, *Breast* 8:175–181, 1999.

Holmes MD, Willett WC: Does diet affect breast cancer risk? *Breast Cancer Res* 6(4):170–178, 2004.

Horrobin DF et al: Abnormalities in plasma essential fatty acid levels in women with premenstrual syndrome and with nonmalignant breast disease, *J Nutr Med* 2:259–264, 1991.

Hudson T: Breast cancer–considerations to assist the practitioner in clinical recommendations, *Townsend Letter for Doctors and Patients* 227:2002.

Ingram DM, Hickling C, West L et al: A double-blind randomized controlled trial of isoflavones in the treatment of cyclical mastalgia, *Breast* 11:170–174, 2002.

Iodine relieves pain of fibrocystic breasts, *Medical World News,* January 11, 1988, p 25.

Jasienska G, Thune I: Lifestyle, hormones, and risk of breast cancer, *BMJ* 322 (7286):586–587, 2001.

Kohlmeier L, Simonsen N et al: Adipose tissue trans fatty acids and breast cancer in the European Community Multicenter Study on Antioxidants, Myocardial Infarction, and Breast Cancer, *Cancer Epidemiol Biomarkers Prev* 6:705–710, 1997.

Kollias J, Macmillan RD, Sibbering DM et al: Effect of evening primrose oil on clinically diagnosed fibroadenomas, *Breast* 9:35–36, 2000.

Kushi LJ et al: Intake of vitamins A, C and E and postmenopausal breast cancer, *Am J Epidemiol* 144(2):165–174, 1996.

Lemon HM, Rodriguez-Sierra JF: Timing of breast cancer surgery during the luteal menstrual phase may improve prognosis, *Nebr Med J* 81(4):110–115, 1996.

Lu L: Increased urinary excretion of 2-hydroxyestrone but not 16 -hydroxyestrone in premenopausal women during a soya diet containing isoflavones, *Cancer Res* 60:1299–1305, 2000.

Marshall E: Search for a killer: focus shifts from fat to hormones, *Science* 259:618–621, 1993.

Murkies A: Phytoestrogens and breast cancer in postmenopausal women: a case control study, *Menopause* 7:289–296, 2000.

National Alliance of Breast Cancer Organizations: The diet-breast cancer link, *NABCO News* 11(2):1–2, 1998.

Pashby NL, Mansel RE, Hughes LE et al: A clinical trial of evening primrose oil in mastalgia, *Br J Surg* 68:801–824, 1981.

Pye J et al: Clinical experience of drug treatment for mastalgia, *Lancet* 2:373–377, 1985.

Russo J, Moral R, Balogh GA, Mailo D, Russo IH: The protective role of pregnancy in breast cancer, *Breast Cancer Res* 7(3):131–142, 2005.

Schellenberg R: Treatment for the premenstrual syndrome with *agnus castus* fruit extract: prospective, randomised, placebo controlled study, *BMJ* 322:134–137, 2001.

Stoll BA: Micronutrient supplements may reduce breast cancer risk. How, when and which? *Eur J Clin Nutr* 51:573–577, 1997.

Veer P et al: Tissue antioxidants and postmenopausal breast cancer: the European community multicentre study on antioxidants myocardial infarction and cancer of the breast, *Cancer Epidemiol Biomarkers Prev* 5:441–446, 1996.

We A et al: Tofu and risk of breast cancer in Asian American, *Cancer Epidemiol Biomarkers Prev* 5:901–906, 1996.

Wuttke W, Splitt G, Gorkow C et al: Treatment of cyclical mastalgia: results of a randomised, placebo-controlled, double-blind study [translated from German], *Geburtsh Frauenheilk* 57:569–574, 1997.

CARDIOVASCULAR HEALTH

Arias RD: Cardiovascular health and the menopause: the gynecologist as the patient's interface, *Climacteric* 9(5):6–12, 2006.

Butler J et al: Metabolic syndrome and the risk of cardiovascular disease in older adults, *JACC* 47:1595–1602, 2006.

Clarke R, Armitage J: Vitamin supplements and cardiovascular risk: review of the randomized trials of homocysteine-lowering vitamin supplements, *Semin Thromb Hemost* 26(3):341–348, 2000.

Eikelboom JW, Lonn E, Genest J Jr, Hankey G, Yusuf S: Homocyst(e)ine and cardiovascular disease: a critical review of the epidemiologic evidence, *Ann Intern Med* 131(5):363–375, 1999.

Erasmus U: *Fats that heal, fats that kill*, Vancouver, BC, 1994, Alive Books.

Erden F et al: Ascorbic acid effect on some lipid fractions in human beings, *Acta Vitaminol Enzymol* 7(1):131–138, 1985.

Goode GK, Garcia S, Heagerty AM: Dietary supplementation with marine fish oil improves in vitro small artery endothelial function in hypercholesterolemic patients, *Circulation* 96:2802–2807, 1997.

Greene CM et al: Maintenance of the LDL cholesterol: HDL cholesterol ratio in an elderly population given a dietary cholesterol challenge, *J Nutr* 135:2793–2798, 2005.

Jandak JM et al: Alpha tocopherol: an effective inhibitor of platelet adhesion, *Blood* 73(1):141–149, 1989.

Khan F, Elherik K, Bolton-Smith C et al: The effects of dietary fatty acid supplementation on endothelial function and vascular tone in healthy subjects, *Cardiovasc Res* 59(4):955–962, 2003.

Koumans AK, Wildschut AJ: Nutrition and atherosclerosis: some neglected aspects, *Clin Cardiol* 8:547–551, 1985.

Krumholz HM et al: Lack of association between cholesterol and coronary heart disease mortality and morbidity and all cause mortality in persons older than 70 years, *JAMA* 272(17):1335–1340, 1994.

Morcos NC: Modulation of lipid profile by fish oil and garlic combination, *JNMA* 89:673–678, 1997.

Ness AR et al: Vitamin C status and the blood pressure, *J Hypertens* 14(4):503–508, 1996.

Olsson AG: The antioxidants in the prevention of atherosclerosis, *Curr Opin Cardiol* 12:188–194, 1997.

Paolisso G, Barbagallo M: Hypertension, diabetes mellitus and insulin resistance, *Am J Hypertens* 10:346–355, 1997.

Rimm EB, Stampfer MJ: The role of antioxidants in preventive cardiology, *Curr Opin Cardiol* 12:188–194, 1997.

Sammartino A et al: Osteoporosis and cardiovascular disease: benefit-risk of hormone replacement therapy, *J Endocrinol Invest* 28(10 suppl):80–84, 2005.

Sowers MR et al: Association of intakes of vitamin D and calcium with blood pressure among women, *Am J Clin Nutr* 42:135–142, 1985.

Stringer MD, Gorog PG, Freeman A, Kakkar VV: Lipid peroxides and atherosclerosis, *BMJ* Feb 4;298(6669): 281–284, 1989.

COCCYDYNIA

Hodges SD et al: A treatment and outcomes analysis of patients with coccydynia, *Spine J* 4(2):138–140, 2004.

Maigne JY et al: Causes and mechanisms of common coccydynia: role of body mass index and coccygeal trauma, *Spine* 25(23):3072–3079, 2000.

Maigne JY et al: Instability of the coccyx in coccydynia, *J Bone Joint Surg Br* 82(7):1038–1041, 2000.

Maigne JY et al: Comparison of three manual coccydynia treatments: a pilot study, *Spine* 26(20):E479–E483, 2001.

Maigne JY et al: The treatment of chronic coccydynia with intrarectal manipulation: a randomized controlled study, *Spine* 31(18):E621–E627, 2006.

Polkinghorn BS, Colloca CJ: Chiropractic treatment of coccygodynia via instrumental adjusting procedures using activator methods of chiropractic technique, *J Manipulative Physiol Ther* 22(6):411–416, 1999.

Ryder I, Alexander J: Coccydynia: a woman's tail, *Midwifery* 16(2):155–160, 2000.

CULTURAL CONSIDERATIONS

American Medical Student Association: Cultural competency in medicine (accessed Dec. 2006), http://www.amsa.org/programs/gpit/cultural.cfm.

Berlin EA, Fowkes WC: Teaching framework for cross-cultural care: application in family practice, *West J Med* 139(6):934–938, 1983.

Fadiman A: *The spirit catches you and you fall down: a Hmong child, her American doctors, and the collision of two cultures,* New York, 1997, Farrar, Straus & Giroux.

Isaacs MR, Benjamin MP: *Towards a culturally competent system of care: volume II,* Washington, DC, 1991, CASSP Technical Assistance Center, Georgetown University Child Development Center.

Kavanagh KH, Kennedy PH: *Promoting cultural diversity: strategies for health care professionals,* Newbury Park, CA, 1992, Sage.

Kielich AM, Miller L: Cultural aspects of women's health care, *Patient Care* 30 (16):60–76, 1996.

Kleinman A: *Patients and Healers in the Context of Culture,* University of California Press, Berkeley, CA, 1980.

National Center for Cultural Competence: Developing cultural competence in health care settings, *Pediatr Nurs* 28:133–137, 2002.

Pachter LM: Culture and clinical care: folk illness beliefs and behaviors and their implications for health care delivery, *JAMA* 271(9):690–694, 1994.

Population projections of the United States by age, sex, race, and Hispanic origin: 1995–2050, Bureau of the Census, p25–1130, 1996, US Dept. of Commerce.

Rostand SG: Ultraviolet light may contribute to geographic and racial blood pressure differences, *Hypertension* 30(2 pt 1):150–156, 1997.

Salimbene S: *What language does your patient hurt in?* Amherst, MA, 1995, Amherst Educational Publishing.

Silva JK et al: Ethnic differences in perinatal outcome of gestational diabetes mellitus, *Diabetes Care* 29:2058–2063, 2006.

DIABETES

American Diabetes Association Nutrition Recommendations and Interventions for Diabetes–2006: a position statement of the American Diabetes Association, *Diabetes Care* 29:2140–2157, 2006.

Barinas-Mitchell E et al: Effect of weight loss and nutritional intervention on arterial stiffness in type 2 diabetes, *Diabetes Care* 29:2218–2222, 2006.

Barnard ND et al: A low-fat vegan diet improves glycemic control and cardiovascular risk factors in a randomized clinical trial in individuals with type 2 diabetes, *Diabetes Care* 29:1777–1783, 2006.

Brock DW et al: A high-carbohydrate, high-fiber meal improves endothelial function in adults with the metabolic syndrome, *Diabetes Care* 29:2313–2315, 2006.

Bureau of Statistics–National Diabetes Information Clearinghouse: www.http://diabetes.niddk.nih.gov/dm/pubs/statistics/estimates.htm Dec 2006.

Carr DB et al: Gestational diabetes mellitus increases the risk of cardiovascular disease in women with a family history of type 2 diabetes, *Diabetes Care* 29:2078–2083, 2006.

Halat KM, Dennehy CE: Botanicals and dietary supplements in diabetic peripheral neuropathy, *J Am Board Fam Pract* 16(1):47–57, 2003.

Hamman RF et al: Effect of weight loss with lifestyle intervention on risk of diabetes, *Diabetes Care* 29:2102–2107, 2006.

Jack AM, Keegan A, Cotter MA et al: Effects of diabetes and evening primrose oil treatment on responses of aorta, corpus cavernosum and mesenteric vasculature in rats, *Life Sci* 71(16):1863–1877, 2002.

Keen H et al: Treatment of diabetic neuropathy with gamma linolenic acid, *Diabetes Care* 16:8–13, 1993.

Martin J et al: Chromium picolinate supplementation attenuates body weight gain and increases insulin sensitivity in subjects with type 2 diabetes, *Diabetes Care* 29:1826–1832, 2006.

Orr R et al: Mobility impairment in type 2 diabetes: association with muscle power and effect of tai chi intervention, *Diabetes Care* 29:2120–2122, 2006.

Rekeneire ND et al: Diabetes, hyperglycemia, and inflammation in older individuals: the Health, Aging and Body Composition Study, *Diabetes Care* 29:1902–1908, 2006.

Robinson K et al: Low circulating folate and vitamin B_6 concentrations: risk factors for stroke, peripheral vascular disease, and coronary artery disease. European COMAC Group, *Circulation* 97(5):437–443, 1998.

Van Dam RM et al: Dietary calcium and magnesium, major food sources, and risk of type 2 diabetes in U.S. black women, *Diabetes Care* 29:2238–2243, 2006.

Ziegler D, Gries FA: Alpha-lipoic acid in the treatment of diabetic peripheral and cardiac autonomic neuropathy, *Diabetes* 46(suppl 2):S62–S66, 1997.

DOMESTIC VIOLENCE

King CM: Changing women's lives: The primary prevention of violence against women, *Clinical Issues in Perinatal and Women's Health Nursing* 4(3),1993.

Kyriacou DN, McCabe F, Anglin D et al: Emergency department–based study of risk factors for acute injury from domestic violence against women, *Ann Emerg Med* 31(4):502–506, 1998.

McAfee RE: Physicians and domestic violence. Can we make a difference? *JAMA* 273(22):1790, 1995.

Tjaden P, Thoennes N: Extent, nature, and consequences of intimate partner violence. Findings from the National Violence Against Women Survey, July 2000, NJC 181867.

US Department of Justice, Office of Justice Programs: *Bureau of justice statistics.* Crime characteristics. http://www.ojp.usdoj.gov/bjs/cvict_c.htm#relate Dec 2006.

US Preventive Services Task Force: Screening for family and intimate partner violence: recommendation statement, *Ann Fam Med* 2(2):156–160, 2004.

Zink T, Elder N, Jacobson J, Klostermann B: Medical management of intimate partner violence considering the stages of change: precontemplation and contemplation, *Ann Fam Med* 2(3):231–239, 2004.

Organizations

Community Action Council-Lewis House, Eagan, MN.
Cornerstone, Bloomington, MN.
Domestic Abuse Intervention Project, Duluth, MN.
Domestic Abuse Project, Minneapolis, MN.
Harriet Tubman Center, Minneapolis, MN.
Minnesota Coalition for Battered Women, St. Paul, MN.
National Coalition Against Domestic Violence, Denver, CO.
National Domestic Violence Hotline: 1–800–799–7233 (1–800–799-SAFE).
National Resource Center on Domestic Violence, Harrisburg, PA.

DYSMENORRHEA

Deutch B: Menstrual pain in Danish women correlated with low n-3 polyunsaturated fatty acid intake, *Eur J Clin Nutr* 49:508–516, 1995.

Fontana-Klaiber H, Hogg B: Therapeutic effects of magnesium in dysmenorrhea, *Schweiz Rundsch Med Prax* 79(16):491–494, 1990.

Harel Z et al: Supplementation with omega-3 polyunsaturated fatty acids in the management of dysmenorrhea in adolescents, *Am J Obstet Gynecol* 174(4): 1335–1338, 1996.

Havens CS, Sullivan ND, Tilton P: *Manual of outpatient gynecology*, Boston, 1996, Little, Brown.

Kaplan B et al: Clinical evaluation of a new model of a transcutaneous electrical nerve stimulation device for the management of primary dysmenorrhea, *Gynecol Obstet Invest* 44(4):255–259, 1997.

Klein TA: Office gynecology for the primary care physician, part II. Pelvic pain, vulvar disease, disorders of menstruation, premenstrual syndrome and breast disease, *Med Clin North Am* 80:321–336, 1996.

Kokjohn K, Schmid DM, Triano JJ, Brennan PC: The effect of spinal manipulation on pain and prostaglandin levels in women with primary dysmenorrhea, *J Manipulative Physiol Ther* 15:279–285, 1992.

Lievl NA, Butler LM: A chiropractic approach to the treatment of dysmenorrhea, *J Manipulative Physiol Ther* 13:101–106, 1990.

Mannheimer JS, Whalen E: The efficacy of transcutaneous electrical nerve stimulation in dysmenorrhea, *Clin J Pain* 1(2):75–83, 1985.

Penland J, Johnson P: Dietary calcium and manganese effects on menstrual cycle symptoms, *Am J Obstet Gynecol* 168:1417–1423, 1993.

Proctor M, Farquhar C: Diagnosis and management of dysmenorrhea, *BMJ* 332:1134–1138, 2006.

Rocker I: *Pelvic pain in women: diagnosis and management*, London, 1990, Springer-Verlag.

Thomason PR, Fisher BL, Carpenter PA, Fike GL: Effectiveness of spinal manipulative therapy in treatment of primary dysmenorrhea: a pilot study, *J Manipulative Physiol Ther* 2:140–145, 1979.

Ziaei S, Faghihzadeh S, Sohrabvand F et al: A randomized placebo-controlled trial to determine the effect of vitamin E in treatment of primary dysmenorrhea, *Br J Obstet Gynaecol* 108:1181–1183, 2001.

DYSPAREUNIA

Berman JR, Berman LA, Goldstein I: Female sexual dysfunction: past, present, and future, *Med Aspects Hum Sex* 1(5):15–20, 1998.

Canavan TP, Heckman CD: Dyspareunia in women: breaking the silence is the first step toward treatment, *Postgrad Med* 108:2, 2000.

Derogatis LR, Melisaratos N: The DSFI: a multidimensional measure of sexual functioning, *J Sex Marital Ther* 5:244–281, 1979.

Heim LJ: Evaluation and differential diagnosis of dyspareunia, *Am Fam Physician* 63:1535–1544, 1551–1552, 2001.

Jamieson DJ, Steege JF: The prevalence of dysmenorrhea, dyspareunia, pelvic pain, and irritable bowel syndrome in primary care practices, *Obstet Gynecol* 87(1): 55–58, 1996.

Meana M, Binik YM: Painful coitus: a review of female dyspareunia, *J Nerv Ment Dis* 182:264–272, 1994.

Meana M, Binik YM, Khalifé S, Cohen D: Biopsychosocial profile of women with dyspareunia, *Obstet Gynecol* 90:583–589, 1997.

Peckham BM, Maki DG, Patterson IJ et al: Focal vulvitis: a characteristic syndrome and cause of dyspareunia: features, natural history and management, *Am J Obstet Gynecol* 154:855–864, 1986.

Petok WD: A practical approach to evaluating female sexual dysfunction, *OBG*, March 1999, pp 68–78.

Rhodes JC et al: Hysterectomy and sexual functioning, *JAMA* 282(20):1934–1941, 1999.

Rocker I: *Pelvic pain in women: diagnosis and management*, London, 1990, Springer-Verlag.

Rosen RC, Leiblum SR: Treatment of sexual disorders in the 1990's: an integrated approach, *J Consult Clin Psychol* 63:877–890, 1995.

Steege JF: Dyspareunia and vaginismus, *Clin Obstet Gynecol* 27:750–759, 1984.

Steege JF et al: Chronic pelvic pain in women: toward an integrative model, *Obstet Gynecol Surv* 48:95, 1993.

Travel J, Simons D: *The trigger point manual*, Baltimore, 1983, Williams & Wilkins.

ENDOMETRIOSIS

Bland J: *Medical applications of clinical nutrition*, New Canaan, CT, 1983, Keats.

Davis SI, Blanck HM, Hertzberg VS et al: Menstrual function among women exposed to polybrominated biphenyls: a follow-up prevalence study, *Environ Health* 4:15, 2005.

Hamann I: Effects of isoflavonoids and other plant derived compounds on the hypothalamus-pituitary-thyroid hormone axis, *Maturitas*, Aug 8, 2006.

Hart R: Unexplained infertility, endometriosis, and fibroids, *BMJ* 327:721–724, 2003.

Havens CS, Sullivan ND: *Manual of outpatient gynecology*, Philadelphia, 2002, Lippincott Williams & Wilkins.

Heidenry C: *Making the transition to a macrobiotic diet*, New York, 1988, Avery.

Kresch JA: In Martin DC, editor: *An atlas of endometriosis*, London 1993, Grower Medical Publishing.

Lee JR, Hanley J, Hopkins V: *What your doctor may not tell you about premenopause*, New York, 1999, Warner Books.

Paolisso G, Barbagallo M: Hypertension, diabetes mellitus and insulin resistance, *Am J Hypertens* 10:346–355, 1997.

Perper MM, Nezhat F, Goldstein H, Nezhat CH, Nezhat C: Dysmenorrhea is related to the number of implants in endometriosis patients, *Fertil Steril* 63:500–503, 1995.

Phelps J: Headliners: reproductive health: effects of organochlorine compounds on menstrual cycles, *Environ Health Perspect* 113(7):A455, 2005.

Reid G, Jass J, Sebulsky MT, McCormick JK: Potential uses of probiotics in clinical practice, *Clin Microbiol Rev* 16(4):658–672, 2003.

Ripps BA, Martin DC: Focal pelvic tenderness, pelvic pain and dysmenorrhea in endometriosis, *J Reprod Med* 36:470–472, 1991.

Rock JA: Endometriosis and pelvic pain, *Fertil Steril* 60:950–951, 1993.

Shames RL: Nutritional management of stress-induced dysfunction, *ANSR Applied Nutritional Science Reports,* November 2003.

Shills ME: *Modern nutrition in health and disease*, Philadelphia, 1998, Lea & Febiger.

Shills ME et al: *Modern nutrition in health and disease*, ed 9, Baltimore, 1999, Williams & Wilkins.

Smith WL, Langenbach R: Why there are two cyclooxygenase isozymes, *J Clin Invest* 107(12):1491–1495, 2001.

Steege JF et al: Chronic pelvic pain in women: toward an integrative model, *Obstet Gynecol Surv* 48:95, 1993.

Sutton C: The role of laparoscopic surgery in the treatment of minimal to moderate endometriosis, *Gynaecol Endosc* 2:131–133, 1993.

Taber CW: *Taber's cyclopedic medical dictionary*, FA Davis.

Ventolini G, Horowitz GM, Long R: Endometriosis in adolescence: a long-term follow-up fecundability assessment, *Reprod Biol Endocrinol* 3:14, 2005.

Waller KG, Shaw RW: GnRH analogues for the treatment of endometriosis: long-term follow-up, *Fertil Steril* 59:511–515, 1993.

FEMALE ATHLETE TRIAD

De La Torre DM, Snell BJ: Use of the preparticipation physical exam in screening for the female athlete triad among high school athletes, *J Sch Nurs* 21 (6):340–345, 2005.

Drinkwater BL, Bruemner B, Chesnut CH 3rd: Menstrual history as a determinant of current bone density in young athletes, *JAMA* 263(4):545–548, 1990.

Drinkwater BL, Nilson K, Chesnut CH 3rd et al: Bone mineral content of amenorrheic and eumenorrheic athletes, *N Engl J Med* 311(5):277–281, 1984.

Gabel KA: Special nutritional concerns for the female athlete, *Curr Sports Med Rep* 5(4):187–191, 2006.

Gidwani GP: Amenorrhea in the athlete, *Adolesc Med* 10(2):275–290, 1999.

Iglesias EA, Coupey SM: Menstrual cycle abnormalities: diagnosis and management, *Adolesc Med* 10(2):255–273, 1999.

Loucks AB, Horvath SM: Athletic amenorrhea: a review, *Med Sci Sports Exerc* 17 (1):56–72, 1985.

Nichols JF et al: Prevalence of the female athlete triad syndrome among high school athletes, *Arch Pediatr Adolesc Med* 160(2):137–142, 2006.

Otis CL: Exercise-associated amenorrhea, *Clin Sports Med* 11(2):351–362, 1992.

Sabatini S: The female athlete triad, *Am J Med Sci* 322(4):193–195, 2001.

Theintz G et al: Longitudinal monitoring of bone mass accumulation in healthy adolescents: evidence for a marked reduction after 16 years of age at the level of the lumbar spine and femoral neck in female subjects, *J Endocrinol Metab* 75(4):1060–1065, 1992.

Torstveit MK, Sundgot-Borgen J: The female athlete triad exists in both elite athletes and controls, *Med Sci Sports Exerc* 37(9):1449–1459, 2005.

Warren MP, Perlroth NE: The effects of intense exercise on the female reproductive system, *J Endocrinol* 170(1):3–11, 2001.

Yurth EF: Physical medicine and rehabilitation: female athlete triad, *West J Med* 162(2):149–150, 1995.

FIBROIDS

Adamson GD: Treatment of uterine fibroids: current findings with gonadotropin-releasing hormone agonists, *Am J Obstet Gynecol* 166(2):746–751, 1992.

Hamann I: Effects of isoflavonoids and other plant derived compounds on the hypothalamus-pituitary-thyroid hormone axis, *Maturitas*, Aug 8, 2006.

Hart R: Unexplained infertility, endometriosis, and fibroids, *BMJ* 327:721–724, 2003.

Lark SM: *Dr. Susan Lark's heavy menstrual flow & anemia self help book*, Berkeley, 1996, Celestial Arts.

Northrup C: *Women's bodies, women's wisdom. Creating physical and emotional health and healing*, New York, 1998, Bantam Books.

Paolisso G, Barbagallo M: Hypertension, diabetes mellitus and insulin resistance, *Am J Hypertens* 10:346–355, 1997.

Shills ME et al: *Modern nutrition in health and disease*, ed 9, Baltimore, 1999, Williams & Wilkins.

Singh A et al: Effect of insulin-like growth factor-type 1 (IFG-I) and insulin on the secretion of sex hormone binding globulin and IGF-I binding protein (IBP-I) by human hepatoma cells, *J Endocrinol* 124(2):R1–3, 1990.

Smith WL, Langenbach R: Why there are two cyclooxygenase isozymes, *J Clin Invest* 107(12):1491–1495, 2001.

Steege JF et al: Chronic pelvic pain in women: toward an integrative model, *Obstet Gynecol Surv* 48:95, 1993.

Storlien LH et al: Fish oil prevents insulin resistance induced by high fat feeding in rats, *Science* 237:885–888, 1987.

Strehl FE: *Internist* 39(9):969–973 1998.

Warshowsky A, Oumano E: *Healing fibroids: a doctor's guide to a natural cure*, New York, 2002, Simon and Schuster.

Zavaroni I et al: Hyperinsulinemia, obesity and syndrome X, *J Intern Med* 235::51–56, 1994.

FIBROMYALGIA

Abraham GE, Flechas JD: Management of fibromyalgia: rationale for the use of magnesium and malic acid, *J Nutr Med* 3:49–59, 1992.

Belch JF, Hill A: Evening primrose oil and borage oil in rheumatologic conditions, *Am J Clin Nutr* 71(suppl):352S–356S, 2000.

Caterina R, Liao JK, Libby P: Fatty acid modulation of the endothelial activation, *Am J Clin Nutr* 71(suppl):213S–223S, 2000.

Cevik R et al: Hypothalamic-pituitary-gonadal axis hormones and cortisol in both menstrual phases of women with chronic fatigue syndrome and effect of depressive mood on these hormones, *BMC Musculoskelet Disord* 5:47, 2004.

Chilton-Lopez T et al Metabolism of gammalinolenic acid in human neutrophils, *Am Associat Immunologists*, 2941–2947, 1996.

Crofford LJ, Appleton BE: Complementary and alternative therapies for fibromyalgia, *Curr Rheumatol Rep* 3(2):147–156, 2001.

Ernst E, Chrubasik S: Phyto-antiinflammatories: a systematic review of randomized, placebo controlled, double-blind trials, *Complementary and Alternative Therapies for Rheumatic Diseases* 26(1):13–27, 2000.

Fisher B, Harbige L: Effect of omega 6 lipid-rich borage oil feeding on immune function in healthy humans, *Biochem Soc Trans* 25:343S, 1997.

Gupta A, Silman AJ: Psychological stress and fibromyalgia: a review of the evidence suggesting a neuroendocrine link, *Arthritis Res Ther* 6(3):98–106, 2004.

Huff L, Brady D: *Instant access to chiropractic guidelines and protocols*, St Louis, 2005, Elsevier Mosby.

Joe LA, Hart LL: Evening primrose oil in rheumatiod arthritis, *Ann Pharmacother* 27(12):1475–1477, 1993.

Leventhal L, Boyce E, Zurier R: Treatment of rheumatoid arthritis with gamma-linolenic acid, *Ann Intern Med* 119:867–873, 1993.

Neeck G, Crofford LJ: Neuroendocrine perturbations in fibromyalgia and chronic fatigue syndrome, *Rheum Dis Clin North Am* 26(4):927–1002, 2000.

Russell IJ, Michalek JE, Flechas JD, Abraham GE: Treatment of fibromyalgia syndrome with Super Malice: a randomized, double-blind, placebo-controlled pilot study, *J Rheumatol*, 22:953–958, 1995.

Young Z, Floyd DL, Loeber G, Tong L: Structure of a closed form of human malic enzyme and implications for catalytic mechanism, *Nature Struct Biol* 7:251–257, 2000.

Zurier R, Rosetti R, Jacobson E et al: Gamma linolenic acid treatment of rheumatoid arthritis. A randomized placebo-controlled trial, *Arthritis Rheumatology* 39 (11):1808–1817, 1996.

INCONTINENCE

Chuang YC et al: Botulinum toxin treatment of urethral and bladder dysfunction, *J Formos Med Assoc* 102(1):5–11, 2003.

Emmons S, Otto L: Acupuncture for overactive bladder: a randomized controlled trial, *Obstet Gynecol* 106:138–143, 2005.

Glazer HI: Long term follow-up of dysesthetic vulvodynia patients after completion of successful treatment by surface electromyography assisted pelvic floor muscle rehabilitation, *J Reprod Med* 45:798–801, 2000.

Hisashi H et al: Acupuncture on clinical symptoms and urodynamic measurements in spinal-cord-injured patients with detrusor hyperreflexia, *Urologia Internationalis* 65:190–195, 2000.

Hoyte P, Barbieri RL: Urinary incontinence and overactive bladder syndrome: management, *ACP Medicine Online* (accessed June 7, 2006), http://www.medscape.com/viewarticle/534298.

Kegel AM: Physiologic therapy for urinary stress incontinence, *JAMA* 146: 915–917, 1951.

More ways to stay dry, *Harvard Women's Health Watch* 5(7):2–3, 1997.

Perry JD, Hullett MS, Bollinger JR: EMG biofeedback treatment of incontinence and other disorders of the pelvic musculature. Presented at the Meeting of the Biofeedback Society of America, Colorado Springs, CO, March 25–28, 1988.

Rowe JW: The NIH Consensus Development Panel: urinary incontinence in adults, *JAMA* 26:612–685, 1989.

Walters MD: Steps in evaluating the incontinent woman, *Contemp Obstet Gynecol* 37:9, 1992.

INFECTIONS

Avorn J et al: Reduction of bacteriuria and pyuria using cranberry juice, *JAMA* 272 (8):588–590, 1994.

Burger O et al: A high molecular mass constituent of cranberry juice inhibits *Helicobacter pylori* adhesion to human gastric mucus, *FEMS Immunol Med Microbiol* 29(4):295–301, 2000.

Clarke-Pearson DL, Dawood MY: *Green's gynecology: essentials of clinical practice*, ed 4, Boston, 1990, Little, Brown.

Farber KS, Barnett ED, Bolduc GR: Antibacterial activity of garlic and onions: a historical perspective, *Pediatr Infect Dis J* 12(7):613–614, 1993.

Fidel PL et al: Systemic cell mediated immune reactivity in women with recurrent vulvovaginal candidiasis, *J Infect Dis* 168:1458, 1993.

Fleet JC: New support for a folk remedy: cranberry juice reduces bacteriuria and pyuria in elderly women, *Nutr Rev* 52(5):168–170, 1994.

Fleury FJ: Adult vaginitis, *Clin Obstet Gynecol* 24:407, 1981.

Goodfriend R: Reduction of bacteriuria and pyuria using cranberry juice, *JAMA* 272(8):588–590, 1994.

Haverkorn MJ, Mandigers J: Reduction of bacteriuria and pyuria using cranberry juice, *JAMA* 272(8):590, 1994.

Holmes KK: Human ecology and behavior and sexually transmitted bacterial infections, *Proc Natl Acad Sci U S A* 91(7):2448–2455, 1994.

Hopkins WJ, Heisey DM, Jonler M et al: Reduction of bacteriuria and pyuria using cranberry juice, *JAMA* 272(8):588–589, 1994.

McGregor JA, Hammill HA: Contraceptive choices for women with medical problems: contraception and sexually transmitted disease: interactions and opportunities, *Am J Obstet Gynecol* 168(suppl):2033, 1993.

Petrin D, Delgaty K, Bhatt R, Garber G: Clinical and microbiological aspects of *Trichomonas* vaginalis, *Clin Microbiol Rev* 11(2):300–317, 1998.

Raz R, Stamm W: A controlled trial of intravaginal estrio in postmenopausal women with recurrent urinary tract infections, *NEJM* 329(11):753–756, 1993.

Reid G, Burton J, Devillard E: The rationale for probiotics in female urogenital healthcare, *Med Gen Med* 6(1):49, 2004.

Reid G, Jass J, Sebulsky MT, McCormick JK: Potential uses of probiotics in clinical practice, *Clin Microbiol Rev* 16(4):658–672, 2003.

Roberts CW, Walker W, Alexander J: Sex-associated hormones and immunity to protozoan parasites, *Clin Microbiol Rev* 14(3):476–488, 2001.

Saavedra M, Taylor B, Lukacs N, Fidel PL Jr: Local production of chemokines during experimental vaginal candidiasis, *Infect Immun* 67(11):5820–5826, 1999.

Sweet RL: Bacterial vaginosis: new approaches for the treatment of bacterial vaginosis, *Am J Obstet Gynecol* 169(suppl):479, 1993.

INFERTILITY

Abma JC, Chandra A, Mosher WD et al: Fertility, family planning, and women's health: new data from the 1995 National Survey of Family Growth, *Vital Health Stat* 23(19):1–114, 1997.

Baird DD, Wilcox AJ: Cigarette smoking associated with delayed conception, *JAMA* 253(20):2979–2983, 1985.

Barbieri RL et al: *Reproductive endocrinology—physiology, pathophysiology, and clinical management*, ed 4, Philadelphia, 1999, WB Saunders, p 588.

Cahill DJ, Wardle PG: Management of infertility, *BMJ* 325(7354):28–32, 2002.

Centers for Disease Control and Prevention: 2002 assisted reproductive technology success rates. In *National summary and fertility clinic reports*, Atlanta, 2002, Centers for Disease Control and Prevention.

Clarke CA: In vitro fertilization-some comparative aspects, *J R Soc Med* 83(4):214–218, 1990.

Davis SI et al: Menstrual function among women exposed to polybrominated biphenyls: a follow-up prevalence study, *Environ Health* 4:15, 2005.

Di Micco et al: The role of d-dimer as first marker of thrombophilia in women affected by sterility: implications in pathophysiology and diagnosis of thrombophilia induced sterility, *J Transl Med* 2:38, 2004.

Faddy MJ, Gosden RG, Gougeon A et al: Accelerated disappearance of ovarian follicles in mid-life: implications for forecasting menopause, *Hum Reprod* 7(10):1342–1346, 1992.

Havens CS, Sullivan ND: *Manual of outpatient gynecology*, ed 4, Philadelphia, 2002, Lippincott Williams & Wilkins.

Kovacs GT, Newman GB, Henson GL: The postcoital test: what is normal? *BMJ* 1(6116):818, 1978.

Petrozza JC: The role of diagnostic laparoscopy in evaluation of infertility, *Infertil Reprod Med Clin North Am* 8:327–335, 1997.

Shephard BD, Shephard CA: *The complete guide to women's health*, ed 2, New York, 1990, Plume.

Toft G et al: Fertility in four regions spanning large contrasts in serum levels of widespread persistent organochlorines: a cross-sectional study, *Environ Health* 4:26, 2005.

Vitzthum VJ, Spielvogel H, Thornburg J: Interpopulational differences in progesterone levels during conception and implantation in humans, *Proc Natl Acad Sci U S A* 101(6):1443–1448, 2004.

Watson A, Vandekerckhove P, Lilford R et al: A meta-analysis of the therapeutic role of oil soluble contrast media at hysterosalpingography: a surprising result? *Fertil Steril* 61(3):470–477, 1994.

MENOPAUSE

AACE Menopause Guidelines Revision Task Force: American Association of Clinical Endocrinologists medical guidelines for clinical practice for the diagnosis and treatment of menopause, *Endocr Pract* 12(3):315–337, 2006.

Alexandersen P et al: The long term impact of 2–3 years of hormone replacement therapy on cardiovascular mortality and atherosclerosis in healthy women, *Climacteric* 9(2):108–118, 2006.

Baeksgaard L, Andersen KP, Hyldstrup L: Calcium and vitamin D supplementation increases spinal BMD in healthy, postmenopausal women, *Osteoporosis Int* 8(3):255–260, 1998.

Brenner PF: The menopause, *West J Med* 136(3):211–219, 1982.

Brown GM: Light, melatonin and the sleep-wake cycle, *J Psychiatry Neurosci* 19(5): 345–353, 1994.

Burg MA et al: Treatment of menopausal symptoms in family medicine settings following the Women's Health Initiative findings, *J Am Board Fam Med* 19(2): 122–131, 2006.

Cabot S: *Smart medicine for menopause*, New York, 1995, Avery.

Chenoy R et al: Effect of oral gamma linolenic acid from evening primrose oil on menopausal flushing, *BMJ* 308(6927):501–503, 1994.

Cyr M, Calon F, Morissette M, Di Paolo T: Estrogenic modulation of brain activity: implications for schizophrenia and Parkinson's disease, *J Psychiatry Neurosci* 27(1):12–27, 2002.

Czekalla J, Gastpar M, Hubner WD, Jager D: The effect of hypericum extract on cardiac conduction as seen in the electrocardiogram compared to that of imipramine, *Pharmacopsychiatry* 30(suppl 2):86–88, 1997.

Darbinyan V, Kteyan A, Panossian A, Garielian E, Wikman G, Wagner H: Rhodiola rosea in stress induced fatigue: a double blind cross over study of a standardized extract, *Phytomedicine* 7:85–89, 2000.

Egyed A, Pentek Z, Magyar Z: Effect of hormone replacement therapy on the mammographic density of the female breast, *Magy Onkol* 49(4):319–325, 2005.

Erasmus U: *Fats that heal, fats that kill*, Vancouver, BC, 1994, Alive Books.

Eskenazi B, Warner M, Marks AR et al: Serum dioxin concentrations and age at menopause, *Environ Health Perspect* 113(7):858–862, 2005.

Ettinger B: When is it appropriate to prescribe postmenopausal hormone therapy? *Menopause* 13(3):404–410, 2006.

Feig SA, Hynote E, Speight N, Magaziner A, Miranda RA, Schachter MB: Summary of the American College for Advancement in Medicine May 2005 Conference: Menopause, Andropause: Power in Transition, *Evid Based Complement Alternat Med* 2(3):413–419, 2005.

Gaster B, Holroyd J: St. John's wort for depression: a systematic review, *Arch Intern Med* 160(2):152–156, 2000.

Gokhale L, Sturdee DW, Parsons AD: The use of food supplements among women attending menopause clinics in the West Midlands, *J Br Menopause Soc* 9 (1):32–35, 2003.

Heikkinen J et al: A 10 year follow up of postmenopausal women on long term continuous combined hormone replacement therapy: update of safety and quality of life findings, *J Br Menopause Soc* 12(3):115–125, 2006.

Henderson VW: The neurology of menopause, *Neurologist* 12(3):149–159, 2006.

Hubner WD, Lande S, Podzuweit H: Hypericum treatment of mild depressions with somatic symptoms, *J Geriatr Psychiatry Neurol* 7(suppl 1):S12–S14, 1994.

Huntley AL, Ernst E: Systematic review of herbal medicinal products for the treatment of menopausal symptoms, *Menopause* 10(5):465–476, 2003.

Janse A et al: The old lady who liked liquorice: hypertension due to chronic intoxication in a memory-impaired patient, *Neth J Med* 63(4):149–150, 2005.

Johnson PE: *Manganese in health and disease*, Boca Raton, FL, 1994, CRC Press.

Kegel AM: Physiologic therapy for urinary stress incontinence, *JAMA* 146:915–917, 1951.

Komar VV, Kit SM, Sischuk LV, Sischuk VM: Effect of Rhodiola rosea on the human mental activity, *Pharmaceutical J* 36(4):62–64, 1981.

Lee JR, Hopkins V: *What your doctor may not tell you about menopause*, New York, 1996, Warner Books.

Lie JH: Evolving approaches in the treatment of menopausal symptoms, *Obstet Gynecol* 108(1):4–5, 2006.

Linde K et al: St. John's wort for depression-an overview and meta-analysis of randomised clinical trials, *BMJ* 313(7052):253–258, 1996.

Maslova LV, Kondratev BI, Maslov LN, Lishmanov IB: The cardioprotective and antiadrenergic activity of an extract of Rhodiola rosea in stress, *Eksp Klin Farmakol* 57(6):61–63, 1994.

Miller RA: DHEA brass ring or red herring? *J Am Geriatr Soc* 45(11):1402–1403, 1997.

Nachtigall LE et al: Complementary and hormonal therapy for vasomotor symptom relief: a conservative clinical approach, *J Obstet Gynaecol Can* 28(4): 279–289, 2006.

Naftolin F et al: The cellular effects of estrogens on neuroendocrine tissues, *J Steroid Biochem* 30(1–6):195–207, 1988.

Nagata C et al: Decreased serum cholesterol concentration is associated with high intake of soy products in Japanese men and women, *J Nutr* 128:203–213, 1998.

Palan PR et al: Effects of menopause and hormone replacement therapy on serum levels of coenzyme Q_{10} and other lipid soluble antioxidants, *Biofactors* 25(1–4):61–66, 2005.

Pataccchioli FR et al: Menopause, mild psychological stress and salivary cortisol: influence of long term hormone replacement therapy, *Maturitas* 55(2):150–155, 2006.

Prior JC: Progesterone as a bone-trophic hormone, *Endocrine Reviews* 11(2): 386–398, 1990.

Raz R, Stamm W: A controlled trial of intravaginal estrio in postmenopausal women with recurrent urinary tract infections, *NEJM* 329(11):753–756, 1993.

Resnick SM et al: Effects of combination estrogen plus progestin hormone treatment on cognition and affect, *J Clin Endocrinol Metab* 91(5):1802–1810, 2006.

Reuse C et al: Menopause: where are we three years beyond WHI? *Rev Med Suisse* 2(53):467–470, 2006.

Rosano GM, Vitale C, Tulli A: Managing cardiovascular risk in menopausal women, *Climacteric* 9(5):19–27, 2006.

Salpeter SR: Meta-analysis: effect of hormone-replacement therapy on components of the metabolic syndrome in postmenopausal women, *Diabetes Obes Metab* 8(5): 538–554, 2006.

Sarrel PM: Sexuality and menopause, *Obstet Gynecol* 75(suppl 4):26–30S, 1990.

Sestak I et al: Influence of hormone replacement therapy on tamoxifen induced vasomotor symptoms, *J Clin Oncol* 24(24):3991–3996, 2006.

Soffa VM: Alternatives to hormone replacement for menopause, *Alternative Therapies* 2(2):34–39, 1996.

Spasov AA, Wikman GK, Mandrikov VB, Mironova IA, Neumoin VV: A double blind, placebo controlled pilot study of the stimulating and adaptogenic effect of Rhodiola rosea SHR-5 extract on the fatigues of students caused by stress during an examination period with a repeated low dose regimen, *Phytomedicine* 7(2):85–89, 2000.

Stuenkel C, Barrett-Connor E: Hormone replacement therapy: where are we now? *West J Med* 171(1):27–30, 1999.

Sultenfuss SW, Sultenfuss TJ: *A woman's guide to vitamins, minerals and alternative healing*, ed 2, Chicago, 1999, NTC/Contemporary Books.

Tamimi RM et al: Combined estrogen and testosterone use and risk of breast cancer in postmenopausal women, *Arch Intern Med* 166(14):1483–1489, 2006.

Taylor M: Alternatives to conventional hormone replacement therapy, *Compr Ther* 23(8):514–532, 1997.

Tsavachidou D, Liebman MN: Modeling and simulation of pathways in menopause, *J Am Med Inform Assoc* 9(5):461–471, 2002.

Valenti G: DHEA replacement therapy for human aging: a call for perspective, *Alcohol Clin Exp Res* 9(4):71–72, 1997.

Vaya J et al: Antioxidant constituents from licorice roots: isolation, structure elucidation and antioxidant capacity for LDL oxidation, *Free Radic Biol Med* 23(2):302–313, 1997.

Yen SSC, Morales AJ, Khorram O: Replacement of DHEA in aging men and women. Department of Reproductive Medicine, University of California-San Diego.

Youngkin EQ, Davis MS: *Women's health: a primary care clinical guide*, ed 2, Stamford, CT, 1998, Appleton & Lange.

MENORRHAGIA

Barrington JW, Bowen-Simpkins P: The levonorgestrel intrauterine system in the management of menorrhagia, *Br J Obstet Gynaecol* 104:614–616, 1997.

Chen BH, Giudice LC: Dysfunctional uterine bleeding, *West J Med* 169(5):280–284, 1998.

Cooke I, Lethaby A, Farquhar C, Cochrane Collaboration, editors: Antifibrinolytics for heavy menstrual bleeding, *Cochrane Library*, Issue 1, Oxford Update Software, 1999.

Crosignani PG et al: Levonorgestrel-releasing intrauterine device versus hysteroscopic endometrial resection in the treatment of dysfunctional uterine bleeding, *Obstet Gynecol* 90:257–263, 1997.

Dockery CJ, Sheppard B, Daly L, Bonnar J: The fibrinolytic enzyme system in normal menstruation and excessive uterine bleeding and the effect of tranexamic acid, *Eur J Obstet Gynaecol Reprod Biol* 24:309–318, 1987.

Eldred JM, Thomas EJ: Pituitary and ovarian hormone levels in unexplained menorrhagia, *Obstet Gynecol* 84:775–778, 1994.

Hallberg L, Hogdahl A, Nilsson L, Rybo G: Menstrual blood loss-a population study: variation in different ages and attempts to define normality, *Acta Obstet Gynecol Scand* 45:320–351, 1966.

Haynes PJ, Anderson AB, Turnbull AC: Patterns of menstrual blood loss in menorrhagia, *Res Clin Forums* 1:73–78, 1979.

Irvine GA, Campbell-Brown MB, Lumsden MA et al: Randomised comparative trial of the levonorgestrel intrauterine system and norethisterone for the treatment of idiopathic menorrhagia, *Br J Obstet Gynaecol* 105:592–598, 1998.

Janssen CA, Scholten PC, Heintz AP: A simple visual assessment technique to distinguish between menorrhagia and normal menstrual blood loss, *Obstet Gynaecol* 85:977–982, 1995.

Kadir RA, Economides DL, Sabin CA, Owens D, Lee CA: Frequency of inherited bleeding disorders in women with menorrhagia, *Lancet* 261:485–489, 1998.

Lahteenmaki P et al: Open randomised study of use of levonorgestrel releasing intrauterine system as an alternative to hysterectomy, *BMJ* 316:1122–1126, 1998.

Lethaby A, Augood C, Duckitt K, Cochrane Collaboration, editors: Nonsteroidal anti-inflammatory drugs for heavy menstrual bleeding, *Cochrane Library*, Issue 1, Oxford Update Software, 1999.

Lethaby A, Irvine G, Cameron I: Cochrane Collaboration, editors: Cyclical progestagens for heavy menstrual bleeding, *Cochrane Library*, Issue 1, Oxford Update Software, 1999.

Osei J, Critchley H: Menorrhagia, mechanisms and targeted therapies, *Curr Opin Obstet Gynecol* 17(4):411–418, 2005.

Prentice A: Medical management of menorrhagia, *BMJ* 319(7221):1343–1345, 1999.

Russell RM: The vitamin A spectrum: from deficiency to toxicity, *Am J Clin Nutr* 71(4):878–884, 2000.

Smith SK, Abel MH, Kelly RW, Baird DT: Prostaglandin synthesis in the endometrium of women with ovular dysfunctional uterine bleeding, *Br J Obstet Gynaecol* 88:434–442, 1981.

Warner PE et al: Menorrhagia: measured blood loss, clinical features, and outcome in women with heavy periods: a survey with follow-up data, *Am J Obstet Gynecol* 192(6):2093–2095, 2005.

OSTEOPOROSIS

Bhambani M et al: Plasma ascorbic acid concentrations in osteoporotic outpatients, *Br J Rheumatol* 31(2):142–143, 1991.

Calvo MS, Park YK: Changing phosphorus content of the US diet: potential for adverse effects on bone, *J Nutr* 126:1168s–1180s, 1996.

Cooper C et al: Dietary protein intake and bone mass in women, *Calcified Tissue International* 58:320–325, 1996.

Epstein S: Update of current therapeutic options for the treatment of postmenopausal osteoporosis, *Clin Ther* 28(2):151–173, 2006.

Free-Graves J et al: Manganese status of osteoporotics and age matched healthy women, *FASEB J* 4:A777, 1990.

Gambacciani M et al: Effects of combined low doses of the isoflavones derivative ipriflavone and estrogen replacement on bone mineral density and metabolism in postmenopausal women, *Maturitas* 28:75–81, 1997.

Gur A, Sarac AJ, Nas K, Cevik R: The relationship between educational level and bone mineral density in postmenopausal women, *BMC Fam Pract* 5:18, 2004.

Hoover PA et al: Postmenopausal bone mineral density: relationship to calcium intake, calcium absorption, residual estrogen, body composition and physical activity, *Can J Pharm* 74:911–917, 1996.

Isenbarger DW, Chapin BI: Current pharmacologic options for prevention and treatment, *Osteoporosis* 101(1):129–142, 1997.

Kim DH, Vaccaro AR: Osteoporotic compression fractures of the spine; current options and considerations for treatment, *Spine J* 6(5):479–487, 2006.

Krall EA, Dawson-Hughes B: Walking is related to bone density and rates of bone loss, *Am Med J* 96:20–26, 1994.

Kulenovic I, Rasic S, Kulenovic E: Osteoporosis: current trends in diagnosis and management, *Bos J Med Sci* 6(1):24–28, 2006.

Lukert BJ et al: Menopausal bone loss is partially regulated by dietary intake of vitamin D, *Calcified Tissue International* 51:173–179, 1992.

Matkovic V et al: Timing of peak bone mass in Caucasian females and its implication for the prevention of osteoporosis. Inference from a cross-sectional model, *J Clin Invest* 93(2):799–808, 1994.

Mortensen L, Charles P: Bioavailability of calcium supplements and the effect of vitamin D: comparisons between milk, calcium carbonate, and calcium carbonate plus vitamin D, *Am J Clin Nutr* 63:354–357, 1996.

New SA et al: Nutritional influence on bone mineral density: a sectional study, *Am J Clin Nutr* 65:1831–1839, 1997.

Prince RL: Diet and the prevention of osteoporotic fractures, *N Engl J Med* 337 (10):670–676, 1997.

Prior JC: Progesterone as a bone-trophic hormone, *Endocrine Reviews* 11(2):386–398, 1990.

Salamon LM et al: Determinants of premenopausal bone mineral density: the interplay of genetic and lifestyle factors, *J Bone Miner Res* 11(10):1557–1564, 1996.

Sammartino A et al: Osteoporosis and cardiovascular disease: benefit-risk of hormone replacement therapy, *J Endocrinol Invest* 28(suppl 10):80–84, 2005.

Scopacasa R et al: Calcium supplementation suppresses bone resorption in early postmenopausal women, *Calcified Tissue International* 62:8–12, 1998.

Sinaki M et al: Efficacy of non-loading exercises in prevention of vertebral bone loss in postmenopausal women: a controlled trial, *Mayo Clin Proc* 64:762–769, 1989.

Suleimann S et al: Effect of calcium intake and physical activity level on bone mass and turnover in healthy, white, postmenopausal women, *Am J Clin Nutr* 63: 72–79, 1997.

Theintz G et al: Longitudinal monitoring of bone mass accumulation in healthy adolescents: evidence for a marked reduction after 16 years of age at the level of the lumbar spine and femoral neck in female subjects, *J Endocrinol Metab* 75(4):1060–1065, 1992.

Toss G: Effect of calcium intake vs other lifestyle factors on bone mass, *J Intern Med* 231:181–186, 1992.

Yasar L et al: Effect of misoprostol on bone mineral density in women with postmenopausal osteoporosis. Prostaglandins and other lipid mediators, *Mediat* 79(3–4):199–205, 2006.

PELVIC INFLAMMATORY DISEASE

Centers for Disease Control and Prevention: Sexually transmitted diseases treatment guidelines 2002, *MMWR Recomm Rep* 51(RR-6):1–78, 2002.

Clarke-Pearson DL, Dawood MY: *Green's gynecology: essentials of clinical practice*, ed 4, Boston, 1990, Little, Brown.

Farber KS, Barnett ED, Bolduc GR: Antibacterial activity of garlic and onions: a historical perspective, *Pediatr Infect Dis J* 12(7):613–614, 1993.

Hillis SE et al: Delayed care of pelvic inflammatory disease as a risk factor for impaired fertility, *Am J Obstet Gynecol* 168:1503, 1993.

McCormack WM: Pelvic inflammatory disease, *N Engl J Med* 330(2):115–119, 1994.

Ness RB, Hillier SL, Kip KE: Bacterial vaginosis and risk of pelvic inflammatory disease, *Obstet Gynecol* 104(4):761–769, 2004.

Ness RB, Hillier SL, Kip KE: Douching, pelvic inflammatory disease, and incident gonococcal and chlamydial genital infection in a cohort of high-risk women, *Am J Epidemiol* 161(2):186–195, 2005.

Reyes I, Abbuhl S: Pelvic inflammatory disease, e-medicine, (accessed Feb 8, 2007), http://www.emedicine.com/emerg/topic410.htm.

Rosenberg MJ et al: Barrier contraceptives and sexually transmitted diseases in women: a comparison of female dependent methods and condoms, *Am J Public Health* 82:669–674, 1992.

Safrin S et al: Long term sequelae of acute pelvic inflammatory disease: a retrospective cohort study, *Am J Obstet Gynecol* 166:1300, 1992.

Scholes D et al: Vaginal douching as a risk factor for acute pelvic inflammatory disease, *Obstet Gynecol* 81:601, 1993.

Westrom L, Eschenbach D: Chapter 58. In Holmes K et al, editors: *Sexually transmitted diseases*, ed 3, New York, 1999, McGraw-Hill.

Westrom L, Joesoef R, Reynolds G et al: Pelvic inflammatory disease and fertility. A cohort study of 1,844 women with laparoscopically verified disease and 657 control women with normal laparoscopic results, *Sex Transm Dis* 19(4):185–192, 1992.

PERIMENOPAUSE

Boers GH et al: Unique efficiency of methionine metabolism in premenopausal women may protect against vascular disease in the reproductive years, *J Clin Invest* 72(6):1971–1976, 1983.

Chenoy R et al: Effect of oral gamolenic acid from evening primrose oil on menopausal flushing, *BMJ* 308(6927):501–503, 1994.

De Souza MC et al: A synergistic effect of a daily supplement for 1 month of 200 mg magnesium plus 50 mg vitamin B_6 for the relief of anxiety-related premenstrual symptoms: a randomized, double-blind, crossover study, *J Womens Health Gend Based Med* 9(2):131–139, 2000.

Gokhale L, Sturdee DW, Parsons AD: The use of food supplements among women attending menopause clinics in the West Midlands, *J Br Menopause Soc* 9(1): 32–35, 2003.

Huntley AL, Ernst E: Systematic review of herbal medicinal products for the treatment of menopausal symptoms, *Menopause* 10(5):465–476, 2003.

Lee JR, Hanley J, Hopkins V: *What your doctor may not tell you about premenopause*, New York, 1999, Warner Books.

Manber R et al: Acupuncture for hot flashes, *Fertil Steril,* September 2006.

Maxson WS, Hargrove JT: Bioavailability of oral micronized progesterone, *Fertil Steril* 44(5):622–626, 1985.

McCarty MF: High-dose pyridoxine as an "anti-stress" strategy, *Med Hypotheses* 54(5):803–807, 2000.

McKinlay SM et al: The normal menopausal transition, *Maturitas* 14:103–115, 1992.

NIH state-of-the-science conference statement on management of menopause-related symptoms, March 21-23, 2005 (accessed October 2006), http://consensus.nih.gov/2005/2005MenopausalSymptomsSOS025html.htm.

North American Menopause Society: Clinical challenges of perimenopause: consensus opinion of the North American Menopause Society, *Menopause* 7: 5–13, 2000.

Northrup C: *The wisdom of menopause: creating physical and emotional health and healing during the change*, New York, 2001, Bantam Books.

Obermeyer CM: Menopause across cultures: a review of the evidence, *Menopause* 7:184–192, 2000.

Paolisso G, Barbagallo M: Hypertension, diabetes mellitus and insulin resistance, *Am J Hypertens* 10:346–355, 1997.

Schmidt PJ et al: Estrogen replacement in perimenopause-related depression: preliminary report, *Am J Obstet Gynecol* 183:414–420, 2000.

Shaw C: The perimenopausal hot flash: epidemiology, physiology and treatments, *Nurse Pract* 2(3):55–65, 1997.

Soares CN et al: Efficacy of estradiol for the treatment of depressive disorders in perimenopausal women: a double-blind, randomized, placebo-controlled trial, *Arch Gen Psychiatry* 58:529–534, 2001.

Stanton MF, Lowenstein FL: Serum magnesium in women during pregnancy while taking contraceptives and after menopause, *J Am Coll Nutr* 6(4):313–319, 1987.

Taylor M: Botanicals: medicines and menopause, *Clin Obstet Gynecol* 44 (4):853–863, 2001.

POLYCYSTIC OVARY SYNDROME

Azziz R et al: The prevalence and features of the polycystic ovarian syndromes in an unselected population, *J Clin Endocrinol Metab* 89:2745–2749, 2004.

Boulman N et al: Increased C-reactive protein levels in polycystic ovarian syndromes: a marker of cardiovascular disease, *J Clin Endocrinol Metab* 89:2160–2165, 2004.

Ehrman DA et al: Prevalence of impaired glucose tolerance and diabetes in females with polycystic ovarian syndrome, *Diabetes Care* 22:141–146, 1999.

Glueck CJ: Incidence and treatment of the metabolic syndrome in newly referred female with confirmed polycystic ovarian syndrome, *Metabolism* 52:908–915, 2003.

Hart et al: Definition, prevalence and symptoms of polycystic ovaries and polycystic ovarian syndrome, *Best Prac Res Clin Obstet Gynaecol* 18:671–683, 2004.

Hopkinson ZE, Sattar N, Fleming R, Greer IA: Polycystic ovarian syndrome: the metabolic syndrome comes to gynecology, *BMJ* 317(7154):329–332, 1998.

Insulin Resistance Syndrome Task Force: American College of Endocrinology position statement on the insulin resistance syndrome, *Endocr Pract* 9:236–252, 2003.

Mavropoulos JC, Yancy WS, Hepburn J, Westman EC: The effects of a low-carbohydrate, ketogenic diet on the polycystic ovary syndrome: a pilot study, *Nutr Metab* (Lond) 2:35, 2005.

Nestler JE: A direct effect of hyperinsulinemia on serum sex hormone binding globulin levels in obese women with polycystic ovary syndrome, *J Clin Endocrinol Metab* 72:83–89, 1991.

Nestler JE: Insulin resistance effects on sex hormones and ovulation in the polycystic ovary syndrome. In Reaven G, Laws A, editors: *Contemporary endocrinology: insulin resistance*, Totowa, NJ, 1999, Humana Press.

Nestler JE, Jakubowicz DJ: Lean women with PCOS respond to insulin reduction with decreases in ovarian P450 c17 alpha activity and serum androgens, *J Clin Endocrinol Metab* 82:4075–4079, 1997.

Pierpoint T et al: Mortality of females with polycystic ovarian syndromes at long term follow up, *J Clin Epidemiol* 51:581–586, 1998.

Rebar R, Judd HL, Yen SS, Rakoff J, Vandenberg G, Naftolin F: Characterization of the inappropriate gonadotropin secretion in polycystic ovary syndrome, *J Clin Invest* 57(5):1320–1329, 1976.

Sheehan MT: Polycystic ovarian syndrome: diagnosis and management, *Clin Med Res* 2(1):13–27, 2004.

Tarik A et al: Ovarian stockpiling in polycystic ovary syndrome, infertility, and the combined use of rosiglitazone and metformin, *Diabetes Care* 29:2330–2331, 2006.

PREGNANCY; PREGNANCY—LABOR AND DELIVERY; PREGNANCY—POSTPARTUM

Agarwal A et al: Role of oxidative stress in female reproduction, *Reprod Biol Endocrinol* 3:28, 2005.

Alfonso DD: Missing pieces—a study of postpartum feelings, *Birth and the Family Journal* 4(4):159, 1977.

American Academy of Pediatrics, American College of Obstetricians and Gynecologists: *Guidelines for perinatal care*, Washington, DC, 1997 Authors.

American Diabetes Association: Gestational diabetes mellitus (position statement), *Diabetes Care* 26(suppl 1):S103–S105, 2003.

Beck CT: Screening methods for postpartum depression, *J Obstet Gynecol Neonatal Nurs* 24:308–312, 1995.

Beck CT: The effects of postpartum depression on maternal-infant interaction: a meta-analysis, *Nurs Res* 44(5):298–304, 1995.

Bjorklund K et al: Sonographic assessment of symphyseal joint distention during pregnancy and post partum with special reference to pubic pain, *Acta Obstet Gynecol Scand* 78(2):125–130, 1999.

Bjorklund K et al: Symphyseal distention in relation to serum relaxin levels and pelvic pain in pregnancy, *Acta Obstet Gynecol Scand* 79(4):269–275, 2000.

Brown JE: *Nutrition and pregnancy: a complete guide from preconception to postdelivery*, Los Angeles, 1998, Contemporary.

Buck GM et al: Maternal fish consumption and infant birth size and gestation: New York State Angler Cohort Study, *Environ Health* 2:7, 2003.

Chibbar R, Miller FD, Mitchell BF: Synthesis of oxytocin in amnion, chorion, and decidua may influence the timing of human parturition, *J Clin Invest* 91(1):185–192, 1993.

Cuilin Z et al: Dietary fiber intake, dietary glycemic load, and the risk for gestational diabetes mellitus, *Diabetes Care* 29:2223–2230, 2006.

Damen L et al: Pelvic pain during pregnancy is associated with asymmetric laxity of the sacroiliac joints, *Acta Obstet Gynecol Scand* 80(11):1019–1024, 2001.

Damen L et al: Does a pelvic belt influence sacroiliac joint laxity? *Clin Biomech (Bristol, Avon)* 17(7):495–498, 2002.

Diakow PR et al: Back pain during pregnancy and labor, *J Manipulative Physiol Ther* 14(2):116–118, 1991.

Esch S, Zachman Z: Adjustive procedures for the pregnant chiropractic patient, *Chiropractic Technique* 3(2):66, May 1991.

Fallon J: *Textbook on chiropractic and pregnancy*, Arlington, VA, 1994, International Chiropractors Association.

Fisher DA: The unique endocrine milieu of the fetus, *J Clin Invest* 78(3):603–611, 1986.

Folkers K, Ellis J: Successful therapy with vitamin B_6 and vitamin B_2 of the carpal tunnel syndrome and need for determination of the RDAs for vitamins B_6 and B_2 for disease states, *Ann N Y Acad Sci* 585:295–301, 1990.

Francis S: *Acupuncture and herbs for obstetrics for mother and infant: a text for professionals and lay persons*, Los Angeles, 1981, Mandala Press.

Hassid P: *Textbook for childbirth educators*, Hagerstown, MD, 1978, Harper & Row.

Kieffer EC et al: Health behaviors among women of reproductive age with and without a history of gestational diabetes mellitus, *Diabetes Care* 29:1788–1793, 2006.

Kinnunen TI, Luoto R, Gissler M, Hemminki E, Hilakivi-Clarke L: Pregnancy weight gain and breast cancer risk, *BMC Women's Health* 4:7, 2004.

Leboyer F: *Birth without violence*, ed 10, New York, 1977, Alfred A. Knopf.

Lewis PJ: Pain in the hand and wrist. Pyridoxine supplements may help patients with carpal tunnel syndrome, *BMJ* 310(6993):1534, 1995.

Lumeng L et al: Adequacy of vitamin B₆ supplementation during pregnancy: a prospective study, *Am J Clin Nutr* 29(12):1376–1383, 1976.

Main KM et al: Human breast milk contamination with phthalates and alterations of endogenous reproductive hormones in infants three months of age, *Environ Health Perspect* 114(2):270–276, 2006.

Mayer-Davis EJ et al: Breast feeding and risk for childhood obesity: does maternal diabetes of obesity status matter? *Diabetes Care* 29:2231–2237, 2006.

Metzger BE, Coustan DR: Proceedings of the Fourth International Workshop-Conference on Gestational Diabetes Mellitus, *Diabetes Care* 21(suppl 2): B1–B167, 1998.

Nutrition during pregnancy, ACOG patient education publication ap001, Washington, DC, 1995, ACOG.

Occhipinti M: Fitness programming for post-natal mothers, *AFPA Fitness* (accessed August 29, 2006), www.afpafitness.com/articles/postnat.htm.

Odent M: *Birth reborn*, New York, 1984, Random House.

O'Mara PO: *Having a baby naturally: the* Mothering Magazine *guide to pregnancy and childbirth*, New York, 2003, Simon & Schuster.

Osborne-Sheets C: *Pre- and perinatal massage therapy*, San Diego, 1998, Body Therapy Associates.

Osmack M: Diastasis recti, prevention and treatment, *Fit 4 two* (accessed August, 29, 2006), http://www.fit4two.ca/Diastasis Recti.htm.

Oxorn H: *Human labor and birth*, ed 5, Connecticut, 1986, Appleton-Century-Crofts.

Phillips CJ: *Hands of love, seven steps to the miracle of birth*, St Paul, MN, 2001, New Dawn Publishing.

Rush D: Periconceptional folate and neural tube defect, *Am J Clin Nutr* 59 (suppl):511s–516s, 1994.

Russo J, Moral R, Balogh GA, Mailo D, Russo IH: The protective role of pregnancy in breast cancer, *Breast Cancer Res* 7(3):131–142, 2005.

Sahakian V, Rouse D, Sipes S, Rose N, Niebyl J: Vitamin B₆ is effective therapy for nausea and vomiting of pregnancy: a randomized, double-blind placebo-controlled study, *Obstet Gynecol* 78(1):33–36, 1991.

Schoellner C et al: Pregnancy-associated symphysis damage from the orthopedic viewpoint–studies of changes of the pubic symphysis in pregnancy, labor and postpartum, *Z Orthop Ihre Grenzgeb* 139(5):458–462, 2001.

Senechal PK: Symphysis pubis separation during childbirth, *J Am Board Fam Pract* 7(2):141–144, 1994.

Snow RE, Neubert AG: Peripartum pubic symphysis separation: a case series and review of the literature, *Obstet Gynecol Surv* 52(7):438–443, 1997.

Stillerman E: *Mother massage: a handbook for relieving the discomforts of pregnancy*, New York, 1992, Dell.

Tulchinsky D, Korenman SG: The plasma estradiol as an index of fetoplacental function, *J Clin Invest* 50(7):1490–1497, 1971.

Watanabe M, Meeker CI, Gray MJ, Sims EA, Solomon S: Secretion rate of aldosterone in normal pregnancy, *J Clin Invest* 42(10):1619–1631, 1963.

Youngkin EQ, Davis MS: *Women's health: a primary care clinical guide*, ed 2, Stamford, CT, 1998, Appleton & Lange.

PREMATURE OVARIAN FAILURE

Bakalov V et al: Ovarian failure, e-medicine, May 23, 2005 (accessed October 2006), http://www.emedicine.com/med/topic1700.htm.

Fenichel P et al: Prevalence, specificity and significance of ovarian antibodies during spontaneous premature ovarian failure, *Hum Reprod* 12(12):2623–2628, 1997.

Goswami D, Conway G: Premature ovarian failure, *Hum Reprod Update* 11 (4):391–410, July 2005.

Grosdemouge I, Bachelot A, Lucas A, Baran N, Kelly PA, Binart N: Effects of deletion of the prolactin receptor on ovarian gene expression, *Reprod Biol Endocrinol* 1:12, 2003.

Hoek A, Schoemaker J, Drexhage HA: Premature ovarian failure and ovarian autoimmunity, *Endocr Rev* 18(1):107–134, 1997.

Hundscheid RD et al: Imprinting effect in premature ovarian failure confined to paternally inherited fragile X premutations, *Am J Hum Genet* 66(2):413–418, 2000.

Kalantaridou SN et al: Treatment of autoimmune premature ovarian failure, *Hum Reprod* 14(7):1777–1782, 1999.

Kalantaridou SN et al: Premature ovarian failure, endothelial dysfunction and estrogen-progestogen replacement, *Trends Endocrinol Metab* 17(3):101–109, 2006.

Koh JM, Kim CH, Hong SK: Primary ovarian failure caused by a solvent containing 2-bromopropane, *Eur J Endocrinol* 138(5):554–556, 1998.

Ledent C et al: Premature ovarian aging in mice deficient for Gpr3, *Proc Natl Acad Sci U S A* 102(25):8922–8926, 2005.

Nelson LM, Bakalov VK: Mechanisms of follicular dysfunction in 46, XX spontaneous premature ovarian failure, *Endocrinol Metab Clin North Am* 32(3):613–637, 2003.

Taylor AE et al: A randomized, controlled trial of estradiol replacement therapy in women with hypergonadotropic amenorrhea, *J Clin Endocrinol Metab* 81 (10):3615–3621, 1996.

PREMENSTRUAL SYNDROME (PMS)

Abraham GE: Nutritional factors in the etiology of the premenstrual tension syndromes, *J Reprod Med* 28(7):446–464, 1983.

Abraham GE, Grewal J: A total dietary program emphasizing magnesium instead of calcium, *J Reprod Med* 35:503–507, 1990.

Abraham GE, Hargrove JT: Effect of vitamin B_6 on premenstrual symptomatology in women with premenstrual tension syndromes: a double blind crossover study, *Infertility* 3(2):155–165, 1980.

Braiden V, Metcalf F: Premenstrual tension among hysterectomized women, *J Psychosom Obstet Gynaecol* 16:145–151, 1995.

Budeiri D, Li Wan PA, Dornan JC: Is evening primrose oil of value in the treatment of premenstrual syndrome? *Controlled Clin Trials* 17(1):60–68, 1996.

Casper R: A double blind trial of evening primrose oil in premenstrual syndrome, 2nd International Symposium on PMS, Kiawah Island, September 1987.

Choi PY, Salmon P: Symptom changes across the menstrual cycle in competitive sportswomen, exercisers and sedentary women, *Br J Clin Psychol* 34(pt 3): 447–460, 1995.

Chuong CJ, Dawson EB: Zinc and copper levels in premenstrual syndrome, 62(2): 313–320, 1994.

Chuong CJ, Durgos DM: Medical history in women with premenstrual syndrome, *J Psychosom Obstet Gynaecol* 1691:21–27, 1995.

De Souza MC et al: A synergistic effect of a daily supplement for 1 month of 200 mg magnesium plus 50 mg vitamin B_6 for the relief of anxiety-related premenstrual symptoms: a randomized, double-blind, crossover study, *J Womens Health Gend Based Med* 9(2):131–139, 2000.

Dickerson LM, Mazyck PJ, Hunter MH: Premenstrual syndrome, *Am Fam Physician* 67(8):1743–1752, 2003.

Linde K et al: St John's wort for depression—an overview and meta-analysis of randomized clinical trials, *BMJ* 313:253–258, 1996.

Loch EG, Selle H, Boblitz N: Treatment of premenstrual syndrome with a phyto-pharmaceutical formulation containing *Vitex agnus castus*, *J Womens Health Gend Based Med* 9(3):315–320, 2000.

London RS et al: Efficacy of alpha tocopherol in the treatment of the premenstrual syndrome, *J Reprod Med* 32(6):400–404, 1987.

Martorano JT et al: Differentiating between natural progesterones: clinical implications for premenstrual syndrome management, *Compr Ther* 19(3):96–98, 1993.

Mazyck PJ, Hunter MH: Premenstrual syndrome, *Am Fam Physician* 67 (8):1743–1752, 2003.

Moline ML: Pharmacologic strategies for managing premenstrual syndrome, *Clin Pharm* 12(3):181–196, 1993.

Mortola J: Premenstrual syndrome, *West J Med* 156(6):651, 1992.

Mortola J: A risk-benefit appraisal of drugs used in the management of premenstrual syndrome, *Drug Saf* 10:160–169, 1994.

O'Brien PM: Helping women with premenstrual syndrome, *BMJ* 307:1471–1475, 1993 .

Ocerman P et al: Evening primrose oil as a treatment of the premenstrual syndrome, *Recent Advancements in Clinical Nutrition* 2:404–405, 1986.

Oleson T, Flocco W: Randomized controlled study of premenstrual symptoms treated with ear, hand, and foot reflexology, *Obstet Gynecol* 82:906–911, 1993.

Oyelowo T: Diagnosis and management of premenstrual syndrome in the chiropractic office, *Top Clin Chiro* 4(3):1–10, 1997.

Paolisso G, Barbagallo M: Hypertension, diabetes mellitus and insulin resistance, *Am J Hypertens* 10:346–355, 1997.

Plouffe L et al: Premenstrual syndrome update on diagnosis and management, *Female Patient* 19:53–58, 1994.

Puolakka J et al: Biochemical and clinical effects of treating the premenstrual syndrome with prostaglandin synthesis precursors, *J Reprod Med* 30(3):149–153, 1985.

Rosenstein DL, Tyschon TW, Neimela J: Skeletal muscle intracellular ionized magnesium measured by 31-P-NMR spectroscopy across the menstrual cycle, *J Am Coll Nutr* 14:486–490, 1995.

Rubinow DR: The premenstrual syndrome, new views, *JAMA* 268(14): 1908–1912, 1992.

Schellenberg R: Treatment for the premenstrual syndrome with *agnus castus (Vitex)* fruit extract: prospective, randomised, placebo controlled study, *BMJ* 322:134–137, 2001.

Stolberg M: The monthly malady: a history of premenstrual suffering, *Med Hist* 44(3):301–322, 2000.

Strid J, Jepson R, Moore V et al: Evening primrose oil or other essential fatty acids for premenstrual syndrome [protocol], *Cochrane Library*, 2, Oxford, 2000.

Stude DE: The management of symptoms associated with premenstrual syndrome, *J Manipulative Physiol Ther* 14:209–215, 1991.

Tamborini A, Taurell R: Value of standardized ginkgo biloba extract (EGb 761) in the management of congestive symptoms of premenstrual syndrome [translated from French], *Rev Fr Gynecol Obstet* 88:447–457, 1993.

Van Leusden H: Premenstrual syndrome no progesterone deficiency; premenstrual dysphoric disorder no serotonin deficiency, *Lancet* 346:1443–1444, 1995.

Van Leusden H: Serotonin and premenstrual dysphoric disorder, *Lancet* 347:471, 1996.

Wyatt KM, Dimmock PW, Jones PW, Shaughn, O'Brien PM: Efficacy of vitamin B-6 in the treatment of premenstrual syndrome: systematic review, *BMJ* 318 (7195):1375–1381, 1999.

Yoshimura Y et al: Gonadotropin stimulates ovarian renin-angiotensin system in the rabbit, *J Clin Invest* 93(1):180–187, 1994.

REPRODUCTIVE TRACT MALIGNANCIES

Butterworth CE et al: Improvement in cervical dysplasia associated with folic acid therapy in users of oral contraceptives, *Am J Clin Nutr* 35:73–82, 1982.

Clarke-Pearson DL, Dawood MY: *Green's gynecology: essentials of clinical practice*, ed 4, Boston, 1990, Little, Brown.

Colditz GA et al: Increased green and yellow vegetable intake and lowered cancer deaths in an elderly population, *Am J Clin Nutr* 1:32–36, 1985.

Cvetkovic D: Early events in ovarian oncogenesis, *Reprod Biol Endocrinol* 1:68, 2003.

Goodman MT: Association of soy and fiber consumption with the risk of endometrial cancer, *Am J Epidemiol* 146(4):294–306, 1997.

Havens CS, Sullivan ND, Tilton P: *Manual of outpatient gynecology*, ed 4, Boston, 2002, Little, Brown.

Ho SM: Estrogen, progesterone and epithelial ovarian cancer, *Reprod Biol Endocrinol* 1:73, 2003.

McDonnell BA, Twiggs LB: Hormone replacement therapy in endometrial cancer survivors: new perspectives after the heart and estrogen progestin replacement study and the Women's Health Initiative, *J Low Genit Tract Dis* 10(2):92–101, 2006.

Romney SL et al: Plasma vit C and uterine cervical dysplasia, *Am J Obset Gynecol* 151:976–980, 1985.

Shephard BD, Shephard CA: *The complete guide to women's health*, ed 2, New York, 1990, Plume.

Stratton JF et al: Contributions of BRCA 1 mutations to ovarian cancer, *N Engl J Med* 226:1125–1130, 1997.

Vanderhyden BC, Shaw TJ, Ethier JF: Animal models of ovarian cancer, *Reprod Biol Endocrinol* 1:67, 2003.

Youngkin EQ, Davis MS: *Women's health: a primary care clinical guide*, ed 2, Stamford, CT, 1998, Appleton & Lange.

VULVODYNIA

Amarenco G, Kerdraon J, Bouju P et al: Treatments of perineal neuralgia caused by involvement of the pudendal nerve, *Rev Neurol* (Paris) 153:331–334, 1997.

Beydoun A, Sussman N: Symptomatic treatment of painful neuropathies, *Ob/Gyn Rev Psychiatric Literature* 1:1–18, 2000.

Bohm-Starke N et al: Increased intraepithelial innervation in women with vulvar vestibulitis syndrome, *Gynecol Obstet Invest* 46:256–260, 1998.

Clark TJ, Etherington IJ, Luesley DM: Response of vulvar lichen sclerosus and squamous cell hyperplasia to graduated topical steroids, *J Reprod Med* 44:958–962, 1999.

Davis GD, Hutchison CV: Clinical management of vulvodynia, *Clin Obstet Gynecol* 42(2):221–233, 1999.

Edwards L et al: Childhood sexual and physical abuse. Incidence in patients with vulvodynia, *J Reprod Med* 42:135–139, 1997.

Friedrich EG Jr: Vulvar vestibulitis syndrome, *J Reprod Med* 32:110–114, 1987.

Glazer HI: Long term follow-up of dysesthetic vulvodynia patients after completion of successful treatment by surface electromyography assisted pelvic floor muscle rehabilitation, *J Reprod Med* 45:798–801, 2000.

Glazer HI et al: Treatment of vulvar vestibulitis syndrome with electromyographic biofeedback of pelvic floor musculature, *J Reprod Med* 40:283–290, 1995.

Goetsch MF: Vulvar vestibulitis: prevalence and historic features in a general gynecologic practice population, *Am J Obstet Gynecol* 98:703–706, 1991.

Linqvist EN et al: Is vulvar vestibulitis an inflammatory condition? A comparison of histological findings in affected and healthy women, *Acta Derm Venereol* 77:319–322, 1997.

McDonald JS, Spigos DG: Computed tomography–guided pudendal block for treatment of pelvic pain due to pudendal neuropathy, *Obstet Gynecol* 95:306–309, 2000.

Metts JF: Vulvodynia and vulvar vestibulitis: challenges in diagnosis and management, *Am Fam Physician* 59:1547–1556, 1561–1562, 1999.

Paavonen J: Diagnosis and treatment of vulvodynia, *Ann Med* 27:175–181, 1995.

Powell J, Wojnarowska F: Acupuncture for vulvodynia, *J R Soc Med* 92:579–581, 1999.

Sinha P, Sorinola O, Luesley DM: Lichen sclerosus of the vulva. Long term steroid maintenance therapy, *J Reprod Med* 44:621–624, 1999.

Solomons CC et al: Calcium citrate for vulvar vestibulitis: a case report, *J Reprod Med* 36:879–882, 1991.

Turner ML, Marinoff SC: Pudendal neuralgia, *Am J Obstet Gynecol* 165:1233–1236, 1991.

Westrom LV, Willen R: Vestibular nerve fiber proliferation in vulvar vestibulitis syndrome, *Obstet Gynecol* 91:572–576, 1998.

White G et al: Establishing the diagnosis of vulvar vestibulitis, *J Reprod Med* 42:17–160, 1997.

Index